Updates in Surgery

Vincenzo Mandalà (Ed.)

The Role of Laparoscopy in Emergency Abdominal Surgery

In collaboration with
Antonino Mirabella
Massimo Lupo

Foreword by
Gianluigi Melotti

Springer

Editor
Vincenzo Mandalà
Surgical and Emergencies Department
"Villa Sofia – Cervello" Hospital Trust
Palermo, Italy

In collaboration with
Antonino Mirabella
Massimo Lupo

The publication and the distribution of this volume have been supported by the Italian Society of Surgery

The Editor acknowledges the educational contribution offered by Johnson & Johnson Medical S.p.A.

ISBN 978-88-470-2326-0 e-ISBN 978-88-470-2327-7

DOI 10.1007/978-88-470-2327-7

Springer Milan Dordrecht Heidelberg London New York

Library of Congress Control Number: 2011934377

9 8 7 6 5 4 3 2 1 2012 2013 2014

Cover design: Simona Colombo, Milan, Italy
Typesetting: Graphostudio, Milan, Italy

Springer-Verlag Italia S.r.l. – Via Decembrio 28 – I-20137 Milan
Springer is a part of Springer Science+Business Media (www.springer.com)

This book is dedicated to all Italian Surgeons,
a group to which I proudly belong.

To Elisabetta, Giuliana and Stefano,
and the whole family,
in particular to my father,
my greatest supporter during the beginning of my career.

Foreword

It is my great honor and pleasure to write a preface for this new book from Springer focusing on the role of laparoscopy in emergency surgery.

The work has been edited and supervised by Vincenzo Mandalà, an undisputed expert in modern emergency and trauma surgery, and it presents an excellent overview of the methodologies practiced by the major Italian surgery schools, which have elevated the mini-invasive approach to a principle governing their work and, one might add, their overall approach as clinicians.

The book provides an effective summary of many of the already well-established techniques as well as other, more innovative ones, all of which are employed in compliance with the emergency and safety criteria required by this particular surgical field.

Emergency surgery is one of the most demanding branches of general surgery: time is crucial and any decision must be immediate but nonetheless agreed upon by a multidisciplinary team of surgeons and anesthesiologists able to recognize the benefits of mini-invasive surgery not just during the procedure itself but, above all, during the postoperative period. This is particularly true for the most complex cases. Furthermore, surgeons working in an increasingly technological setting need to be supported by nursing and medical teams familiar with the sophisticated and constantly changing equipment and materials.

In this setting, continuing education plays a crucial role, and books like this one, which summarize techniques, protocols, and evidence, can support surgeons in their decision-making when they are dealing with the various clinical and organizational problems common to both small and large hospitals.

The work–one could even say, the mission–that Vincenzo Mandalà has been carrying out in the most important Italian and international scientific societies makes him an ideal advocate of the approaches underlying this specific surgical field and so well-presented in this volume.

What is certain is that emergency laparoscopy has made the transition and is no longer the last diagnostic step but the first–and, in many cases, the only–therapeutic step.

Thank you Vincenzo for this very fine job!

Rome, October 2011

Gianluigi Melotti
President, Italian Society of Surgery

Preface

Over the last ten years of my professional activity and particularly since 1999 I have been working as head of department at "Villa Sofia-CTO Hospital Trust" in Palermo. The mission of the Hospital Trust is emergency (it has been recognized as a level III leading regional center and a DEA level II, a Department of Emergency and Admission of a high level) and since there was no mini-invasive surgery unit, I decided to make every effort in my daily professional and organizational life towards this new surgical approach. I wanted not only to improve elective laparoscopic advanced surgery, but also to raise the level of emergency surgery by introducing standardized emergency surgery protocols.

Since 1992 I have devoted my professional life to laparoscopic surgery. During a previous experience as the Director of an operative surgery unit in a suburban Hospital (Cefalù Hospital), we had to enhance the use of diagnostic laparoscopy extensively, because of the structural problems and the lack of radiologic imaging modalities such as CT and MR. The laparoscopic approach was, therefore, used for abdominal emergencies, particularly appendicular peritonitis caused by acute appendicitis and perforated ulcers, acute cholecystitis and emergencies of the abdominal wall.

In that period I realized how important diagnostic laparoscopy was not only for neoplastic problems but also for intra-abdominal peritonitis and for nonspecific abdominal pains that mostly affected young women. I found myself being a pioneer of laparoscopic surgery, a technique which can sometimes ensure therapeutic resolutions with all the benefits that we know.

In 1999, I found in the Villa Sofia hospital the structural strength of a large hospital equipped with spiral CT scanning, MR, angiography (although limited), the possibility of intraoperative blood recuperation and intensive care units. For this reason my main aim was to increase emergency laparoscopic surgery, although I have to admit I encountered strong resistance from senior doctors and inexperience but enthusiasm in younger colleagues.

Peritonitis and other nontraumatic emergencies using a laparoscopic approach were the first to be carried out, but as my older colleagues opposed the use of mini-invasive surgery, especially for hemoperitoneum, I had to dedicate myself to tackling abdominal traumas.

Going through the literature concerning abdominal trauma, I realized that laparoscopy had started to be used much earlier than when it actually emerged as a preferred surgical technique, especially for the most dangerous and neglected field of trauma. Estes, Gazzaniga, Cuschieri and Bercy's experiences in fact go back to the 1970s and 1980s.

The problem was not only the doubts regarding the possible benefits of the laparoscopic approach, but - as several trauma surgeons have highlighted - also *the dilemma to decide when and if a laparotomy has to be carried out.* This was underlined by many authors who stressed that missed injuries and therefore an unacceptable delay in treatment should be considered extremely dangerous for patients. They referred to an axiom: *the first rule for emergency abdominal surgery in general, and in particular for trauma abdominal surgery, is the final treatment of all lesions.*

A more recent analysis, although it is not easy to find and elaborate prospective randomized studies, has highlighted that laparotomy is associated with mortality, morbidity and a series of complications which become unacceptable especially when exploration proves negative or nontherapeutic; therefore, all diagnostic procedures, both invasive and noninvasive, become unavoidable if they can reduce explorations which are uncomfortable and useless. Laparoscopy has, recently, shown that when it is carried out by capable hands it can, indisputably, reduce useless explorative laparotomies in at least 40-60% of trauma cases, in particular, for the peritoneal evaluation of the trajectory in penetrating injuries, for diaphragmatic ruptures both in open or blunt trauma and also for the evaluation of non-active bleeding.

Furthermore, laparoscopy allows the surgeon to wait and provides the possibility of using interventional complementary therapies. It must also be stressed that the percentage rate of missed injuries and delayed treatment has dropped 5-10% in the latest evaluations.

Laparoscopy has reached a wider use also thanks to its therapeutic potential, which in the past only concerned some treatment for hemoperitoneum caused by liver and splenic lesions after blunt trauma and for the identification of peritoneal penetration in penetrating trauma. Recently laparoscopy has been widely used for minor lesions (moderate bleeding of the mesentery or moderate lesions of hollow viscous) especially when the surgeon is expert at advanced laparoscopy surgery.

The therapeutic potential of laparoscopy is even more important for emergency nontraumatic surgery. At the beginning of the 1980s Philippe Mouret also demonstrated the real advantages of laparoscopy in acute appendicitis, adhesiolysis and also in peritonitis caused by perforated ulcers.

In the last ten years, as the methodology has undergone increasing improvement it has been possible to carry out laparoscopy in perforated diverticulitis and small bowel obstruction by adhesion and nonadhesion and the approach to nonspecific abdominal pain. Acute pancreatitis and mesenteric ischemia are still to be taken into consideration.

Of course in very many situations laparoscopy cannot be resolutive, but laparoscopic assisted surgery (tailored minilaparotomy) or hand assisted techniques can prove beneficial. Findings in the literature demonstrate that these two different laparoscopic procedures offer the same advantages as pure laparoscopy.

This book about laparoscopy in abdominal emergencies which we believe is the first of its kind has the purpose of underlining the meaning and the potential of minimally invasive surgery in abdominal emergency in trauma and nontraumatic fields.

I am convinced that this study, which is meant to be a guide for specialists and dedicated surgeons, is principally addressed to young internal and trainee surgeons who are faced with emergencies on a daily basis and may also come up against medicolegal problems when they have to take rapid and effective decisions.

Besides being an easy text for consultation, I hope it can stimulate all colleagues with an interest in these problems. I am strongly convinced that we can meet the challenge of putting together guidelines, protocols and records, in order to standardize topics that are currently only in the planning stage. Finally, I am sure that the ever growing technological innovations together with the technical experience of surgical teams will ensure that today's role of laparoscopy in emergency abdominal surgery will maintain its continual and exponential growth. This will make it a diagnostic and therapeutic strong point in so many decisional algorithms of emergency surgery.

Lastly, I would like to make some acknowledgments: to the board of the governors of the Italian Society of Surgery and its President Professor Melotti, an experienced surgeon in this area, for giving me the opportunity to submit this manuscript on behalf of the Association; to Professor Enrico De Antoni for considering my request years ago; and to all the professors, colleagues and my dear assistants who have actively collaborated in the writing of this book and to the publisher Springer Verlag Italia for the effective book layout, the assistance and the patience during the production of this book.

Palermo, October 2011 **Vincenzo Mandalà**

Contents

Contributors

Ferdinando Agresta Azienda ULSS 19 di Adria, UOC di Chirurgia Generale, Presidio Ospedaliero di Adria, Adria (RO), Italy

Luca Ansaloni General Surgery, Ospedali Riuniti di Bergamo, Bergamo, Italy

Grazia M. Attinà Department of Surgery, "S. Agostino-Estense" New Hospital Modena, Italy

Gianpaolo Balzano Pancreas Unit, Department of Surgical Sciences, San Raffaele Scientific Institute, Milan, Italy

Natalino Bedin Department of General Surgery, Presidio Ospedaliero di Vittorio Veneto, Vittorio Veneto (TV), Italy

Fabio Cesare Campanile General Surgery, Andosilla Hospital, Civita Castellana (VT), Italy

Luciano Casciola Department of Surgery, Division of General, Minimally Invasive and Robotic Surgery, ASL 3 Umbria, "San Matteo degli Infermi" Hospital, Spoleto (PG), Italy

Fausto Catena Department of General Emergency and Transplant Surgery, "S. Orsola-Malpighi" University Hospital, Bologna, Italy

Graziano Ceccarelli Department of Surgery, Division of General, Minimally Invasive and Robotic Surgery, ASL 3 Umbria, "San Matteo degli Infermi" Hospital, Spoleto (PG), Italy

Gianfranco Cocorullo General and Emergency Surgery, University of Palermo, Palermo, Italy

Paolo Colobraro General Surgery, Andosilla Hospital, Civita Castellana (VT), Italy

Francesco Corcione Department of General, Laparoscopic and Robotic Surgery, Azienda Ospedaliera dei Colli Monaldi-Cotugno-CTO, Naples, Italy

Diego Cuccurullo Department of General, Laparoscopic and Robotic Surgery, Azienda Ospedaliera dei Colli Monaldi-Cotugno-CTO, Naples, Italy

Fausto Di Marco Department of General and Emergency Surgery, "Villa Sofia – Cervello" Hospital Trust, Palermo, Italy

Salomone Di Saverio General Emergency and Laparoscopic Surgery, Trauma Surgery Unit, Maggiore Hospital, Bologna, Italy

Federico Famiglietti Digestive and Colorectal Surgery, Centre for Minimally Invasive Surgery, University of Turin, Turin, Italy

Nicola Foti General Surgery, Andosilla Hospital, Civita Castellana (VT), Italy

Boris Franzato General Surgery, "San Giacomo Apostolo" Hospital, Castelfranco Veneto (TV), Italy

Grazia Fusco General Surgery, "San Giacomo Apostolo" Hospital, Castelfranco Veneto (TV), Italy

Gaspare Gulotta General and Emergency Surgery, University of Palermo, Palermo, Italy

Camillo La Barbera Department of Oncologic Sciences Policlinico, Palermo, Italy

Benedetto La Motta Department of General and Emergency Surgery, "Villa Sofia – Cervello" Hospital Trust, Palermo, Italy

Raffaele Landi General Surgery and Laparoscopic Unit, "San Giuliano" Hospital, ASL Na2 Nord, Giugliano (NA), Italy

Gianluca Lanni General Surgery and Laparoscopic Unit, "San Giuliano" Hospital, ASL Na2 Nord, Giugliano (NA), Italy

Massimo Lupo Department of General and Emergency Surgery, "Villa Sofia – Cervello" Hospital Trust, Palermo, Italy

Stefano Mandalà Service de Chirurgie Digestive et Endocrinienne, NHC Hôpitaux Universitaires, Strasbourg, France

Vincenzo Mandalà Department of General and Emergency Surgery, "Villa Sofia – Cervello" Hospital Trust, Palermo, Italy

Domenico Marchi Department of Surgery, "S. Agostino-Estense" New Hospital, Modena, Italy

Gianluigi Melotti Department of Surgery, "S. Agostino-Estense" New Hospital, Modena, Italy

Antonino Mirabella Department of General and Emergency Surgery, "Villa Sofia – Cervello" Hospital Trust, Palermo, Italy

Mario Morino Digestive and Colorectal Surgery, Centre for Minimally Invasive Surgery, University of Turin, Turin, Italy

Alberto Patriti Department of Surgery, Division of General, Minimally Invasive and Robotic Surgery, ASL 3 Umbria, "San Matteo degli Infermi" Hospital, Spoleto (PG), Italy

Nicolò Pecorelli Pancreas Unit, Department of Surgical Sciences, San Raffaele Scientific Institute, Milan, Italy

Micaela Piccoli Department of Surgery, "S. Agostino-Estense" New Hospital, Modena, Italy

Antonio Pinna Head of General Emergency and Transplant Surgery Department, "S. Orsola-Malpighi" University Hospital, Bologna, Italy

Felice Pirozzi Department of General, Laparoscopic and Robotic Surgery, Azienda Ospedaliera dei Colli Monaldi-Cotugno-CTO, Naples, Italy

Gabriele Salvatore General Surgery and Laparoscopic Unit, "San Giuliano" Hospital, ASL Na2 Nord, Giugliano (NA), Italy

Carlo A. Sartori General Surgery, "San Giacomo" Hospital, Castelfranco Veneto, (TV), Italy

Antonio Sciuto Department of General, Laparoscopic and Robotic Surgery, Azienda Ospedaliera dei Colli Monaldi-Cotugno-CTO, Naples, Italy

Carlo Staudacher Head of Department of Surgical Sciences, San Raffaele Scientific Institute, Milan, Italy

Vincenzo Trapani Department of Surgery, "S. Agostino-Estense" New Hospital, Modena, Italy

Annunziato Tricarico Head of General Surgery and Laparoscopic Unit, "San Giuliano" Hospital, ASL Na2 Nord, Giugliano (NA), Italy

Nereo Vettoretto Laparoscopic Surgery Unit, "M. Mellini" Hospital, Chiari (BS), Italy

Diagnostic Laparoscopy in Abdominal Emergencies

1

Ferdinando Agresta, Antonello Mirabella, Natalino Bedin and Vincenzo Mandalà

1.1 Introduction

Acute emergency situations often pose a diagnostic challenge to the general surgeon. The diagnosis is important due to the different pathologic conditions that might be responsible for the acute situation and therefore important for planning the correct abdominal incision or avoiding an unnecessary laparotomy. There are several noninvasive diagnostic procedures – such as ultrasonography and CT scanning – which can be performed along with plain film radiography on patients with an acute abdomen to aid the surgeon in establishing a preoperative diagnosis [1–12]. In experienced hands, which are not always available around the clock in every hospital setting, the results of these methods are quite good, but in general practice they are not completely accurate and conclusive (partly due to the patients' physical limitations, e.g. obesity or massive bowel distension, and partly because, as already stated, they are dependent on operator skills) and they might be time-consuming and expensive (such as CT scanning) [13–15]. Another factor to keep in mind is that nowadays the mean patient age is increasing and, as a consequence, there is an increasing possibility of being confronted with emergency abdominal situations in the elderly with many co-morbidities which complicate not only the therapeutic strategy but the diagnostic approach as well. In the imaginary equilateral triangle which represents the danger signal for every kind of acute abdomen, the diagnostic side of the triangle and the therapeutic side are increasingly tied together by the technique which for over twenty years has been calling the attention of the surgical world: laparoscopy. Once the diagnosis is established, laparoscopy in fact can take a further step in many cases,

F. Agresta (✉)
Azienda ULSS 19 di Adria
UOC di Chirurgia Generale, Presidio Ospedaliero di Adria,
Adria (RO), Italy

V. Mandalà, *The Role of Laparoscopy in Emergency Abdominal Surgery*,

since therapeutic intervention via laparoscopy is possible for a number of these conditions without the need to resort to a laparotomy (OP) [1–12].

1.2 Laparoscopy: Once a Revolution, Still in Evolution

In writing about laparoscopy in a book on emergency surgery, it seems impossible to divide the diagnostic from the therapeutic value of this approach. Therefore, it is a must to analyze how the attitude towards this approach has changed regarding indications, morbidity and the kind of pathologic conditions, based on the available scientific evidence, for wich laparoscopy might be a good alternative to an open approach – both in terms of diagnosis and treatment.

1.3 Indications

The absolute and relative contraindications to laparoscopy in approaching abdominal emergencies are the same as for elective procedures [1, 6, 7, 9]. As for peritonitis, concerns have been raised that the creation of capnoperitoneum in patients with established peritonitis may be detrimental in terms of worsening bacteremia, endotoxemia and severe sepsis, and experimental studies have yielded conflicting data in this regard. In animal models of peritonitis, endotoxemia and the development of intra-abdominal abscesses do not seem to be increased by CO_2 laparoscopy when compared with control groups [15–20]. Over the past few years there has been an increasing number of series on the use of laparoscopy in the treatment of peritonitis which have reported favorable results, especially in the intensive care unit. In this situation in fact diagnostic laparoscopy (DL) has its main indication for unexplained sepsis, systemic inflammatory response syndrome, acute acalculous cholecystitis, mesenteric ischemia and multisystem organ failure [6]. Generally speaking, peritonitis should not be considered a contraindication to laparoscopy and we do agree with the clinical practice guideline drawn up by the European Association for Endoscopic Surgery (EAES): *Changes in systemic inflammatory and anti-inflammatory parameters ... are less pronounced after laparoscopic surgery than conventional surgery. Whether this leads to clinically relevant effects remains to be proven. There is no compelling clinical evidence that specific modifications of the pneumoperitoneum alter immunologic response... presupposing appropriate perioperative measures and hemodynamic stability, there are no contraindication to create a pneumoperitoneum when laparoscopic surgery is applicable in cases of peritonitis* [20]. Last but not least, we support the idea of minimizing post-surgical infection, not only with the use of antibiotic prophylaxis, but also by optimizing the immune response by maintaining homeostasis through nutritional support (especially the via enteral – and the laparascopy assuring a faster GI recovery allows for an earlier enteral feeding!) and reducing surgical trauma (as is done with laparascopy) which consequently reduces the stress response and immune suppression [21].

Prior abdominal surgery or a known malignancy were thought, by many and in the beginning, a direct indication for laparotomy. However, these conditions are no longer considered an absolute contraindication to laparoscopic exploration for emergency situations, provided the possibility of establishing a pneumoperitoneum [1–6].

Lastly, the use of emergency laparoscopy in the pediatric arena has been limited, with contraindications both in terms of local experience and modification and availability of pediatric equipment, i.e. mini-instruments. There has nonetheless been an increasing number of reports of a laparoscopic approach in children with acute abdominal situations, above all with suspicion of acute appendicitis, with good results especially regarding the diagnostic value of laparoscopy [22]. With regard to older patients, it should be born in mind that they tend to present later in the course of their illness and have more non-specific symptoms. In addition, a broader differential diagnosis must be considered in older patients with abdominal pain. Moreover, they often have numerous other conditions that may be responsible for changes in physical status or laboratory parameters. Therefore, the early diagnosis of abdominal complications is a clinical challenge, but it is of the utmost importance because early diagnosis and especially early treatment are the determinant keys of clinical outcome [23, 24]. If there are no absolute contraindications to the approach, laparoscopy might offer a change in diagnosis and treatment, reducing the amount of trauma in patients with "weak" or "border line" general conditions. Generally speaking we no longer consider age (both in the two extreme periods: pediatric and old age) as a contraindication to laparoscopy [23, 24].

1.4 Diagnostic Accuracy

The diagnostic accuracy of laparoscopy is reported with a rate of 89–100% in the international literature [1, 6, 7, 9, 25]. Generally speaking, the most common cause of acute abdominal pain is non-specific abdominal pain (NSAP) (22–44% of the study population), followed by acute appendicitis (15–29%), acute biliary disease (3–10%) and bowel obstruction or diverticulitis in elderly patients. Acute appendicitis represents the cause of surgical intervention in two-thirds of children with acute abdomen. The high diagnostic yield of laparoscopy is important especially in the first two situations: patients with pelvic disease – suspected appendicitis and NSAP, where laparoscopy allows for a more thorough exploration of the abdominal cavity and identification of concomitant diseases than OP. A delay in surgical intervention while further investigations are performed may increase morbidity and prolong hospital stay (average delay period of 6.12 days), especially considering that patients admitted with unclear diagnosis – namely with NSAP – might be old, obese, critically ill and with co-morbid situations (such as diabetes and immunosuppressive therapy) [8–10]. With regard to preoperative imaging, the accuracy of radiography in these diseases reaches 75%, whereas the accuracy of abdominal ultrasound is 60–89%. The CT scan is more accurate (84–98%), but it is not always available in all hospital settings [13–15]. It has been reported in the literature that with an open approach, such as in suspected appendicitis, the accurate on-table diagnosis is missed in up to 14.3% of cases and that the sensitivity for diagnosing normal appendices is low at 51.3%, thus suggesting that almost half of normal appendices might be misdiagnosed as pathologic, with the risk of no further exploration for other pathologic conditions [26].

Another main advantage of laparoscopy is the management of generalized peritonitis, where a better quality of peritoneal washing and an easy cleaning in the deep abdominal areas (such as the rectouterine pouch), as well as minimal destruction of the abdominal wall, can be done [1, 6, 25]. In addition, many patients with acute suppurative peritonitis do not have an obvious perforation, but rather an inflammatory and necrotic zone with edema and abscess formation. Therefore they can be safely treated with drainage near the diseased zone with a broad peritoneal lavage and antibiotic therapy. This procedure may allow for second-stage laparoscopic treatment of the underlying disease, such as a resection of sigmoid diverticula in elective conditions [27].

Even though the level of evidence is not particularly high, the large number of case reports in the literature concerning generally benign rare disease responsible for cases of acute abdomen which might be not correctly diagnosed by laparotomy (and sometimes left in situ with the possibility of a clinical and symptomatic return) has to be taken in consideration.

At the extreme end of the spectrum, diagnostic laparoscopy has been proposed for trauma patients to prevent unnecessary exploratory laparotomies with their associated higher morbidity and cost. A significant number of patients who sustain penetrating trauma to the anterior abdominal wall do not suffer a peritoneal breach. Therefore, proof that penetration has not occurred negates the need for laparotomy. Current diagnostic imaging – such as US and CT – are unable to provide this, due to high false negative rates. Studies of DL for trauma report negative procedures with a range from 17 to 89% (median 57%), with a range concerning negative laparotomies after a false positive DL from 0 to 44 % (median 6%). While most authors have converted to open exploration after a positive DL, some authors have successfully treated the majority of patients (up to 83%) laparoscopically. Laparoscopy is also an excellent modality to evaluate the diaphragm in penetrating thoraco-abdominal injuries. Concerning blunt trauma, although stable patients may undergo diagnostic laparoscopy to exclude relevant injury, its efficacy in this subgroup is still unproven [6, 25].

1.5 Conversion, Morbidity and Mortality

The results of several experiences show the feasibility of DL in abdominal emergencies with acceptable morbidity and mortality rates (0–24% morbidity and 0–4.6% mortality) comparable to those reported for OP. The complications reported are various and different and mainly concern general and local patient conditions, the underlying disease and the technique itself (iatrogenic morbidity such as injury to vascular and parenchymal structures and so on). Since the procedure has been applied to patients with variable disease acuity and operative risk, complications are higher in studies which include sicker patients and the majority of reported deaths are associated with multiple organ failure secondary to sepsis [1, 6, 25].

With regard to conversion, the most frequent causes are the presence of dense adhesions and unclear anatomy, or the lack of skill and experience on the part of the surgeon in facing the single and specific cause of the acute abdomen. What is important to point out is that converted procedures have similar hospital stays compared with open ones [1, 6, 25].

Surgical timing is another relevant issue which influence diagnostic/therapeutic efficacy, conversion, morbidity and mortality: the earlier the better. As shown mainly in acute cholecystitis and perforated gastroduodenal ulcers, the degree of inflammation is strictly related to the time from the onset of symptoms [28–30].

1.6 Treatment Options

Laparascopy offers the possibility of undertaking the same surgical procedures as open surgery, or even scheduling the appropriate medical therapy in the presence of concomitant diseases [1, 6, 7, 9, 25]. The length of surgery is almost equal (and in some cases is undoubtedly shorter) than open surgery, due to improvements in both equipment and the surgeon's learning curve. The time spent for treatment of diseases incidentally found at laparoscopy should be weighed against the economic impact of a missed diagnosis [1, 6, 7, 9, 25].

1.7 Hospital Stay

Although the available evidence seems to be mixed concerning hospital stay after DL (due to several biases), it is becoming increasingly shorter when compared with open and observational controls, and patients experience a faster and uneventful recovery. The reduced length of hospital stay is particularly evident if we do not split the diagnostic value of laparoscopy from its therapeutic one in patients operated on for pelvic disease, small bowel obstruction (SBO) and cholecystitis [1, 6, 7, 9, 25].

1.8 Costs

No evidence exists on the general cost-effectiveness of DL for the acute abdomen. But we do believe that the advantage of laparascopy does not only consist of cosmesis but also of a decrease in operative trauma. So it might be right to say that the costs are balanced by the fact that the laparoscopic procedure reduces the time needed to make the diagnosis and provide treatment, thereby saving money on imaging studies and shorter hospital stay with decreasing morbidity from progressive disease [1, 6, 7, 9, 25]. As a consequence – although the exact economic impact of laparoscopy is difficult to assess, namely if direct costs are taken into account – the earlier patients recover and return to work does benefit society as a whole. Another point to keep in mind: with the already existing equipment, there is no better way to achieve a more cost-effective and full utilization of these facilities than by expanding them to emergency procedures – even if only for a diagnostic purpose.

1.9 The Surgeon

The profile of the surgeon and the surgical team is still a crucial issue. A well-trained and experienced surgeon together with a well-trained team is a necessary prerequisite for laparoscopy – both diagnostic and therapeutic. To undertake emergency laparoscopic operations, the surgeon must be experienced [1, 6, 7, 9, 25]. A possibly small operating theatre, together with the wide variety of therapeutic findings, require a well-trained and experienced surgeon as well as a well-trained surgical team. Good judgment is needed for a timely decision to convert the procedure (and plan a "target" incision) in order not to jeopardize and prolong the attempts to complete the operation laparoscopically. We believe that general surgeons are rapidly rather than gradually becoming experienced in laparoscopy, especially in those hospital situations where the laparoscopic approach is not confined to elective procedures and where diagnostic laparoscopy has a used and useful role in the acute abdomen. We think that it is in this area where many junior staff, under supervision, might learn the basic insufflation techniques, become used to handling the laparoscope and instruments as well as becoming orientated in the peritoneum and learning how to perform operative techniques, from the simplest to the most advanced [31, 32]. We can say that laparoscopy in emergency situations will not only benefit the patient but will also benefit many trainee surgeons who will be introduced to this general surgical adjunct this way.

The evidence available to date clearly demonstrates the superiority of a laparoscopic approach in various emergency situations (cholecystitis, gastroduodenal perforated ulcers, appendicitis, gynecologic disorders, NSAP: all grade of recommendation A), but laparoscopy offers lesser or unclear benefits in other acute conditions (small bowel obstruction, acute diverticulitis, incarcerated hernias, mesenteric ischemia – grade of recommendation C; abdominal trauma and pancreatitis: grade of recommendation B) [32–40].

Therefore, a policy of laparoscopy for all patients with acute abdominal pain does not seem justified. The initial usage of diagnostic procedures and imaging should aim to identify those patients who probably would not benefit from laparoscopy. On the other hand, it usually carries only minor disadvantages for a patient if a diagnostic laparoscopy has to be converted to an open procedure.

This enabled us to conclude that in the proper setting, laparoscopic emergency is feasible, effective, safe and beneficial for patients to be a part of common surgical practice, as long as adequate training is obtained and proper preparation observed when more advanced procedures are attempted in critically ill patients. Laparoscopy provides a continuous superior diagnostic accuracy as well as wider therapeutic potentials. The diagnostic and therapeutic versatility afforded by the laparoscopic approach avoids extensive preoperative studies, averts delay in operative intervention and minimizes morbidity and shortens postoperative hospitalization. This approach appears to play a crucial role in the diagnostic and therapeutic algorithm for reproductive-age women, obese patients, and in almost every abdominal emergency. We do think that laparoscopy should be incorporated into the general surgeon's armamentarium for the management of patients with acute abdomen as another tool to be used selectively when indicated and, on the grounds of our data and the data reported in the literature, we advocate a wider adoption of laparoscopy and are confident it will become more relevant in common surgical practice, as it is in our own. Laparoscopy, however, must not be used as an alternative to good clinical judgment.

Our algorithm in patients with acute abdomen is as follows: if there are no contraindications to laparoscopy and if informed consent is obtained, in the presence of a well trained surgical team in minimally-invasive surgery we always approach the abdomen with a laparoscope! We do think that every diagnostic laparoscopy is a spared nontherapeutic laparotomy and it is not rhetoric to state that laparoscopy might at the same time be the last diagnostic step and the first therapeutic act.

References

1. Agresta F, Mazzarolo G, Ciardo LF, Bedin N (2008) The laparoscopic approach in abdominal emergencies: has the attitude changed? A single-center review of a 15-year experience. Surg Endosc 22:1255-1262
2. Balèn E, Herrea M, Tarifa A et al (2005) El papel de la laparoscopia en la cirugìa abdominal urgente (The role of laparoscopy in emergency abdominal surgery). An Sist Sanit Naz 28:81-92
3. Golash V, Willson PD (2005) Early laparoscopy as a routine procedure in the management of acute abdominal pain. A review of 1320 patients. Surg Endosc 19:882-885
4. Kirshtein B, Roy-Shapira A, Lantsberg L et al (2003) The use of laparoscopy in abdominal emergencies. Surg Endosc 17:1118-1124
5. Lam CM, Yuen AW, Chik B et al (2005) Laparoscopic surgery for common surgical emergencies. A population-based study. Surg Endosc 19:774-779
6. Sauerlenad S, Agresta F, Bergamaschi R et al (2006) Laparoscopic for abdominal emergencies. Evidence based guidelines of the European Association for Endoscopic Surgery. Surg Endosc 20:14-29

7. Champault G, Descottes B, Dulucq JL et a (2006) Chirurgie laparoscopique: les recommandations des sociétés savantes spécialisées en 2006, SFCL–SFCE. J Chir (Paris) 143:160-164
8. Warren O, Kinross J, Paraskeva P, Darzi A (2007) Emergency laparoscopy – current best practice. WJES 1:24
9. Domìnguez LC, Sanabria A, Vega V, Osorio C (2011) Early laparoscopy for the evaluation of non specific abdominal pain: a critical appraisal of the evidence. Surg Endosc 25:10-18
10. Morino M, Pellegrino L, Castagna E et al (2006) Acute nonspecific abdominal pain: a randomized, controlled trial comparing early laparoscopy versus clinical observation. Ann Surg 244:881-886
11. Fowler DL Laparoscopy in the Acute Abdomen in Controversies in Laparoscopic Surgery. Assalia A, Gagner M, Schein M Editors – Springer Berlin Heidelkberg 2006, pagg. 45-50.
12. Stefanidis D, Richardson WS, Chang L et al (2009) The role of diagnostic laparoscopy for acute abdominal conditions: an evidence-based review. Surg Endosc 23:16–23
13. Salem TA, Molly RG, O'Dwyer PJ (2005) Prospective study on the role of the CT scan in patients with an acute abdomen. Colorectal Dis 7:460-466
14. Stoker J, van Randen A, Lamèris W, Boermeester MA (2009) Imaging patients with acute abdominal pain. Radiology 253:31-46
15. Andersson RE (2011) Routine ultrasound and limited computed tomography for the diagnosis of acute appendicitis: a surgeon's perspective. World J Surg 35:295-296
16. Fuganti PE, Rodrigues AJ, Rodrigues CJ, Sato M (2006) A comparison of the effects of pneumoperitoneum and laparotomy on natural killer cell mediated cytotoxicity and Walker tumor growth in Wistar rats. Surg Endosc 20:1858-1861
17. Nordentoft T, Bringstrup FA, Bremmelgaard A, Stage JG (2000) Effect of laparoscopy on bacteremia in acute appendicitis: a randomized controlled study. Surg Laparosc Endosc Percutan Tech 10:302-304
18. Strobel O, Wachter D, Werner J et al (2006) Effect of a pneumoperitoneum on systemic cytokine levels, bacterial translocation, and organ complications in a rat model of severe acute pancreatitis with infected necrosis. Surg Endosc 20:1897-1903
19. Moberg AC, Montgomery A (2006) Pneumoperitoneum – Update 2006. In: Neugebauer EAM, Saurland S, Fingerhut A et al (eds) EAES guidelines for endoscopic surgery – twelve years evidence-based surgery in Europe, Springer, Berlin, pp. 87-95
20. Neudecker J, Sauerland S, Neugebauer E et al (2002) The European Association for Endoscopic Surgery clinical practice guideline on the pneumoperitoneum for laparoscopic surgery. Surg Endosc 16:1121-1143
21. Esposito S (2001) Immune system and surgical site infection. J Chemother 13[Suppl 1]:12-16
22. Mattei P (2007) Minimally invasive surgery in the diagnosis and treatment of abdominal pain in children. Curr Opin Pediatr 19:338-343
23. Lyon C, Clark D (2006) Diagnosis of acute abdominal pain in older patients. Am Fam Physician 74:1537-1541
24. Kirshtein B, Perry ZH, Mizrahi S, Lantsberg L (2009) Value of laparoscopic appendectomy in the elderly patient. World J Surg 33:918-922
25. Hon Y; SAGES Guidelines Committee (2008) Diagnostic laparoscopy guidelines. Surg Endosc 22:1353-1383
26. Shum CF, Lim JF, Soo KC, Wong WK (2005) On-table diagnostic accuracy and the clinical significance of routine exploration in open appendectomies. Asian J Surg 28:257-261
27. Stocchi L (2010) Current indications and role of surgery in the management of sigmoid diverticulitis. World J Gastroenterol 16:804-817
28. Gurusamy KS, Samraj K (2006) Early versus delayed laparoscopic cholecystectomy for acute cholecystitis. Cochrane Database Syst Rev 4:CD005440
29. Sanabria AE, Morales CH, Villegas MI (2005) Laparoscopic repair for perforated perpic ulcer disease. Cochrane Database Syst Rev 4:CD004778
30. Bertleff MJ, Lange JF (2010) Laparoscopic correction of perforated peptic ulcer: first choice? A review of literature. Surg Endosc 24:1231-1239

31. Sajid MS, Khan MA, Cheek E, Baig MK (2009) Needlescopic versus laparoscopic appendectomy: a systematic review. Can J Surg 52:129-134
32. Chiu CC, Wei PL, Wang W et al (2006) Role of appendectomy in laparoscopic training. J Laparoendosc Adv Surg Tech 16:113-118
33. Grafen CF, Neuhaus V, Schöb O, Turina M (2010) Management of acute small bowel obstruction for intestinal adhesions: indications for laparoscopy surgery in a community teaching hospital. Langenbecks Arch Surg 395:57-63
34. Zerey M, Sechrist C, Kercher K et al (2007) Laparoscopic management of adhesive small bowel obstruction. Am Surg 73:773-778
35. Cirocchi R, Abraha I, Farinella E et al (2010) Laparoscopic versus open surgery in small bowel obstruction. Cochrane Database Syst Rev 2:CD007511
36. Corneille MG, Steigelman MB, Myers JG et al (2007) Laparoscopic appendectomy is superior to open appendectomy in obese patients. Am J Surg 194:877-880
37. Tzovaras G, Baloyiannis I, Kouritas V et al (2010) Laparoscopic versus open appendectomy in men: a prospective randomized trial. Surg Endosc 24:2987-2992
38. Ghosheh B, Salameh JR (2007) Laparoscopic approach to acute small bowel obstruction: review of 1061 cases. Surg Endosc 21:1945-1949
39. Deeba S, Purkayastha S, Paraskevas P et al (2009) Laparoscopic approach to incarcerated and strangulated inguinal hernias. JSLS 3:327-331
40. Korndorffer JR Jr, Fellinger E, Reed W (2010) SAGES guideline for laparoscopic appendectomy. Surg Endosc 24:757-761

Suggested Readings

Sauerland S, Agresta F, Bergamaschi R, Borzellino G, Budzynski A, Champault G, Fingerhut A, Isla A, Johansson M, Lundorff P (2006) Laparoscopy for abdominal emergencies. Evidence-based guidelines of the European Association for Endoscopic Surgery. Surg Endosc 20:14–29

Agresta F, Ansaloni L, Baiocchi L, Bergamini C, Campanile FB, Carlucci M, Cocorullo G, Corradi A, Franzato B, Lupo M, Mandalà V, Mirabella A, Pernazza G, Piccoli M, Staudacher C, Vettoretto N, Zago M, Lettieri E, Levati A, Pietrini D, Scaglione M, De Masi S, De Placido G, Francucci M, Rasi M, Scaramuzza G, Del Favero AL (2011) Consensus Development Conference of the Società Italiana Chirurgia Endoscopica e nuove tecnologie (SICE); Associazione Chirurghi Ospedalieri Italiani (ACOI); Società Italiana di Chirurgia (SIC); Società Italiana Chirurgia d'Urgenza e Trauma (SICUT), Società Italiana Chirurghi dell'Ospedalità Privata (SICOP) and the European Association for Endoscopic Surgery (EAES). In press

Gastroduodenal Ulcer

2

Antonino Mirabella, Massimo Lupo, Fausto Di Marco
and Vincenzo Mandalà

2.1 Introduction

The advent of more effective and tolerable drugs (H_2 antagonists, proton pump inhibitors, antibiotics for *Helicobacter pylori*, HP, infection) in the treatment of the peptic ulcer has brought about a radical change in the surgical approach to ulcer disease. In fact we can observe an increasing election for minor surgery and a progressive increase in the treatment in emergency for perforating complications. This figure is likely to be attributed on the one hand to the number of surgical indications and on the other to the increasingly widespread use of nonsteroid anti-inflammatory drugs (NSAIDs), especially in the elderly, where surgery has progressively increased in recent years. The peptic ulcer remains the most common cause of gastroduodenal perforation with an incidence ranging from 2% to 10% of the patients with a peptic ulcer [1] and, consequently, the treatment of a perforated peptic ulcer (PPU) remains today the most frequent indication for gastric emergency surgery [2]. The progress of medical treatment, and in particular the radical treatment of HP, has gradually decreased the use of major gastric surgery. Resective treatment (so-called acid-reduction treatment) has decreased as have recurrences of ulcerative disease, and consequently the need for re operation. Considering these conditions the mini-invasive technique, as in other fields, has been adopted to treat a perforated peptic ulcer. This behavior allows us to couple the advantages of laparoscopic surgery (better tolerability for the patient) and the possibility of a definitive treatment of the underlying disease with a relatively simple surgical procedure. After the first report published in 1990 by Mouret et al. [3], which described the technique of the closing of the PPU through an omental

A. Mirabella (✉)
Department of General and Emergency Surgery, "Villa Sofia – Cervello" Hospital Trust,
Palermo, Italy

V. Mandalà, *The Role of Laparoscopy in Emergency Abdominal Surgery*,

patch maintained in situ by fibrin glue in 5 patients, in the same year, Nathanson et al. [4] reported the first laparoscopic surgical treatment of a perforated duodenal ulcer by direct suturing.

2.2 Materials and Methods

We present our experience in the treatment of laparoscopic PPU between April 1999 and December 2010. The results were compared with those present in the literature in the period from 1990 (year of the first work shown on this issue [3, 4]) to 2010. After an electronic search on PubMed, using as key words for the search *laparoscopy*, *repair*, and *perforated peptic ulcer*, more than 100 publications were found. Of these the most relevant are represented by 3 systematic reviews [5-8] and 3 randomized controlled trials (RCTs) [9-11]. During the above mentioned period we performed suture repair for PPU in 98 patients, 65 males and 33 females aged between 23 and 78 years (average 54 years). In 40 patients, the repair of the ulcer was performed with laparoscopic technique (15 females and 25 males, aged between 23 and 75 years, average 50 years). Over the course of time we gradually preferred the mini-invasive treatment to the traditional one. The latter was reserved for patients with unfavorable prognostic factors (state of shock on hospitalization, presence of serious co-morbidity, duration of symptoms >24 h), on the basis of the already known pattern of Boey score [5].

Other contraindications to laparoscopy were previous multiple surgery, patient age >70 years (if associated with poor health) and the limited experience of the surgeon in the field of minimally invasive surgery. The laparoscopic technique we used is the positioning of the patient in Trendelenburg position of 15-20°, with the operator positioned between the legs of the patient. The first optical 10 mm trocar system is positioned in the infra- or supraumbilical cord, generally with an open technique. After the establishment of the pneumoperitoneum (usually at an intra-abdominal pressure of 12 mmHg) and under visual control, the other trocars are positioned, usually 3 and each with a diameter of 5 mm. One trocar is placed in the epigastric zone to separate the liver. The other two trocars are usually positioned respectively in the left and right abdominal quadrant line and above the transverse umbilical.

The first therapeutic act is to the repair the ulcer. In 34 patients we carried out suture repair with reinforcement of the greater omentum; in six patients with friable and edematous lesions we used a technique with omental patches (Figs. 2.1-2.3). In all cases the suture was performed with the intracorporeal technique. Lastly, we performed a thorough and repeated washing of the entire peritoneal cavity with a saline solution, (generally 2-6 L) depending on the seriousness of the peritonitis. At the end of the operation we usually position a single drainage tube in the subhepatic space and near the lesion.

In no patient did we need to revert to open surgery, nor was a re-intervention necessary. We had no mortalities. In one 75-year-old man who had a per-

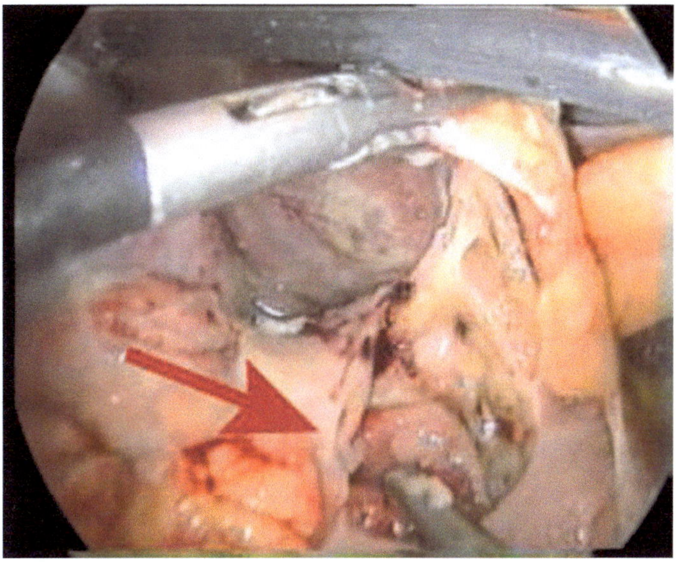

Fig. 2.1 Large perforated piloro-duodenal ulcer, wider than 10 mm in diameter (*red arrow*)

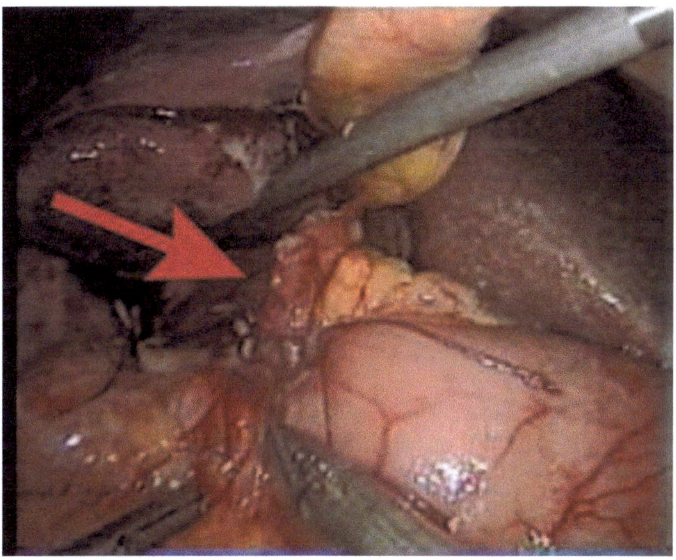

Fig. 2.2 Laparoscopic repair by positioning of omental patch (tension-free technique avoids the risk of stenosis)

forated gastric cancer with early peritoneal cancers (not diagnosed preoperatively), a simple suture repair of the greater omentum was carried out. In 7 patients (>65 years) the laparoscopic biopsy of the lesion was performed

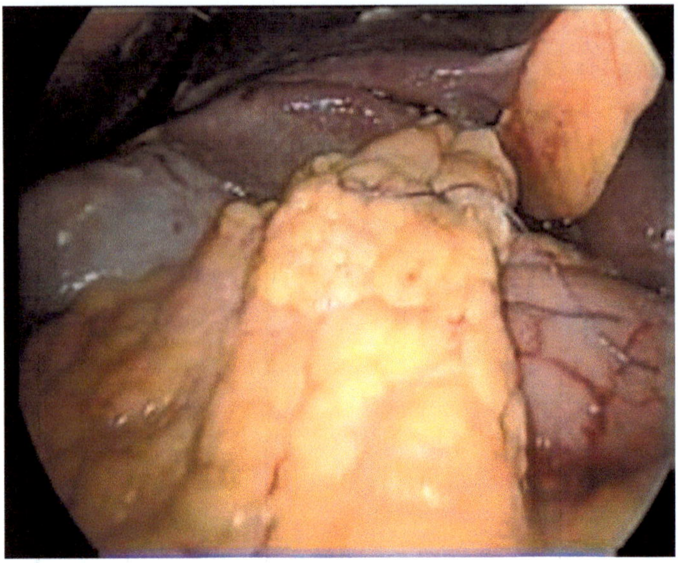

Fig. 2.3 Duodenal ulcer. Laparoscopic repair with reinforcement of the greater omentum

because of a suspected perforated gastric cancer. The results were negative. The average operating times were higher for laparoscopy than for open treatment: 70 min vs. 45 min. There were six cases of serious postoperative complications, consisting of two cases of leakages of sutures with a low-flow fistula which healed spontaneously within 15 days after surgery, one case of gastric bleeding (treated successfully with antacid drugs and repeated blood transfusions) and four cases of lung infections (which responded positively to antibiotic treatment). There was no mortality during the postoperative course, neither in the short or medium term. There were no significant differences between open and laparoscopic surgery in terms of timing of the removal of the nasogastric tube, suspension of parenteral therapy, the resumption of oral diet and the timing of hospitalization (average of 8 days after laparoscopy and 10 days after open treatment).

2.3 Results

2.3.1 Patient Characteristics

A review of the literature reveals a progressive increase in the age of patients with PPU. This data is confirmed by our findings and appears to be due firstly to the effectiveness of anti-ulcer drugs and to the more widespread use of NSAIDs and acetylsalicylic acid in the elderly [2, 12]. As the review by Bertleff and Lange [13] of 54 published articles on the subject over the last twenty years shows, patients with PPU are on average 48 years old. Of these 20% used NSAIDs regularly, a third had a history of peptic ulcer and in 80% of the cases a HP infection was confirmed. The role of a HP infection in the etiopathogenesis of PPU is, however, still not clearly defined, given that the rates of HP infection in the patients who undergo an operation compared to those under medical treatment are identical [12].

2.3.2 Diagnostic Laparoscopy

The clinical suspicion of a perforated peptic ulcer is based on patient history (history of ulcer disease, taking NSAIDs) and on clinical examination (absence or reduction of the hepatic obtuse area during clinical examination). However, sometimes the clinical examination may not be decisive, especially when the leakage from the gastric cavity and the spread of free air in the peritoneum are contained. Generally, laboratory tests are of little use in the acute phase and nonspecific, even if the association of leukocytosis, metabolic acidosis, and hyperamylasemia may be present in the case of duodenal gastric perforation [14]. An indication for surgical exploration is the evidence of sickle air at the base of the right hemidiaphragm on the radiograph (direct radiograph of the abdomen and thoracic bases), associated with a history of peptic ulcer and, on clinical examination, a clear picture of peritonitis [15]. Even if the first instrumental examination used is radiography, this does have limited sensitivity (50-70%) for the confirmation of pneumoperitoneum [16-18].

Experimental studies [16] have shown that to be able to be seen at radiography, the minimum quantity of intraperitoneal gas must be at least 1 mL. Furthermore, the capability of radiography to determine the perforation site is nil [19]. The most reliable examination for the confirmation of free intraperitoneal air is the computed tomography (CT) scan [20, 21]. However, few studies have evaluated the reliability of CT to specify the location of the perforation. Chen et al. [22] in a retrospective study of 14 patients with PPU reported a 100% reliability of a CT scan to determine a pneumoperitoneum, but only 36% in determining the perforation site. In a study of 11 patients with PPU who underwent CT scanning with an oral contrast medium, Fultz et al. [23] correctly localized the lesion in 3 patients (which showed the spreading of contrast medium in the abdomen). In a prospective study of 85 patients with a gastrointestinal perforation (of which 34 with PPU), Hainaux et al. [24] showed an 86% accuracy of CT in specifying the site of the lesion. The extraluminal air bubbles around the stomach (sometimes in the mesentery or near the sigma) or in the duodenum (rarely in the front right pararenal space), a parietal gastric defect or duodenal ulcers, thickening of the mesenteric fat and a segmental thickening of the bowel wall are the most important predictive factors in determining the lesion site [23, 25]. The localization of free peritoneal air around the round ligament [17, 18], the sickle ligament [26] or in the periportal space (the latter considered a far more reliable sign) [27] is evidence of a perforation in the upper gastrointestinal tract.

Today, thanks to the introduction of the modern multidetector CT, the ability to locate the gastrointestinal perforation is high (82-90%) [23, 25], regardless of the use of oral contrast medium, which puts into doubt the real sensitivity benefits concerning the possible adverse effects (risk of complications from aspiration, delay in diagnosis) [28, 29].

Many different studies have reported the use of abdominal ultrasound for the confirmation of free abdominal air. The advantages of this method - the relative ease and repeatability and almost absent invasiveness - justify its use in certain categories of patients such as children and pregnant women, where the risk of exposure to ionizing radiation should always be limited (0.1-4.0 mSv for direct abdominal radiography; 10 mSv for CT) [30]. Although it is able to obtain satisfactory results (sensitivity 85% and specificity 100% in the prospective study by Moriwaky et al. [31]), the technique is unable to reach the level of reliability of a CT and above all is unable to identify the perforation site [32].

In a review by Bertleff and Lange [13] of 54 published articles on the subject over the last twenty years, the diagnosis of a perforation with the presence of free air in the abdomen was possible in 85% of the cases. In addition, as the RCT carried out by the authors themselves shows, in 8 out of 109 patients examined (7%) the laparoscopic diagnosis was different from that of a PPU undertaken prior to the operation [9]. This underlines the importance of the role of laparoscopy, to confirm the diagnosis, to define the location, size and nature of the perforation (a differential diagnosis from other diseases which can cause perforations of the visceral cavity), when the preoperative instrumental investigations have not been positive [8, 10, 33, 34]. For the purpose of a final diagnosis in 93-98% of patients with acute abdomen an exploratory laparoscopy is performed. In 86-100% of cases, mini-invasive treatment is possible during the same operation [33, 35] or, alternatively, a targeted laparotomy based on the evidence seen on the laparoscopic examination may be undertaken.

2.3.3 Selection of Patients/Prognostic Factors

It is clear from the data in the literature that the laparoscopic technique cannot be used in all patients with PPU. In an attempt to pre operatively select the patients suitable for mini-invasive surgery based on objective criteria, several clinical parameters have been defined.

In 1987 Boey and Wong [36] had already established a scale of surgical risk (from 0 to 3) in the treatment of perforated peptic ulcer, according to the presence of three parameters: state of shock on hospitalization (SAP < 90 mmHg), ASA III-V (presence of severe co-morbidity) and duration of symptoms (>24 h). Laparoscopic management would be safe enough for classes 0 and 1, while it should be avoided in those of a higher degree [2, 37]. The conclusions of the meta-analysis by Lau [7] in 2004 favors the use of laparoscopy in PPU in patients with no risk factors (Boey score = 0). In higher risk classes, the conversion rate as well as the mortality rate is significantly higher. This is evident in some studies where there was a high proportion of patients at risk.

Katkhouda et al. [38] present 10 patients in a state of shock (equal to 22% of the total); Robertson et al. [39] present 17 patients (47% of cases) with ASA III-IV, of which 11 underwent laparoscopy. The systematic review by Lunevicius and Morkevicius [8] reached the same conclusions that the laparoscopic approach, which involves an extended operating time compared to the open technique, was not recommended for patients with high risk factors.

Studies by Bertleff et al. [9, 13] have shown how the preoperative classification of risk factors according to the Boey score is highly reliable in deciding the choice of technique to use. However, the limited number of patients present in the study with a high Boey-score (2-3) above all those who underwent laparoscopic treatment make it difficult to find a definitive confirmation of this statement. In conclusion, the authors add that although laparoscopic treatment should represent the treatment of choice in the perforated peptic ulcer, the presence of a Boey score of 3, patient age of 70 years or above and persistent symptoms for more than 24 h, associated with a higher incidence of morbidity and mortality, should be considered contraindications for the use of the mini-invasive technique.

The problem of the duration of the symptoms and a delayed diagnosis is connected to the possibility that the PPU may become an unrecognized peritonitis which is also responsible for a generalized sepsis. In this situation a laparoscopy could play an important role in favoring the migration of bacteria, thanks to the action of CO_2, as has been shown in animal studies [39]. However, such experimental results have not been confirmed by clinical experience. In contrast, a study by Vaidya et al. [40] suggests that the mini-invasive treatment is safe even in patients with peritonitis and a delayed diagnosis. No mortality was recorded out of 31 patients treated laparoscopically for peritonitis caused by PPU and with symptoms for more than 24 h. Several studies have shown the reliability of the Mannheim peritonitis index (MPI score) as a prognostic factor in patients with peritonitis [52, 71]. Patients with a score under 21 have a mortality rate which varies from 0% to 2.3%, in those with higher scores, mortality is nearly 100% [41, 54]. In other experiences the Apache II score has been used to identify patients at risk. The latter is not widely used because many consider it not easily applicable.

Lunevicius and Morkevicius [8] include in the risk factors of a laparoscopy advanced high Boey score, patients over 70 years of age, ApacheII=5 and lastly the surgeon's skill in laparoscopic surgery. However, even these authors underline that a conclusive opinion on the matter cannot be given yet because of the lack of sufficient quantitative data concerning the high risk patients who undergo laparoscopic surgery.

2.3.4 Surgical Technique

Placing the patient in the Trendelenburg position at 15–20° is generally recommended. The surgeon can stand between the patient's legs or at the patient's side. From the review by Berleff and Lange [13] it has been shown that 44% of surgeons prefer the first option (even in our experience this is the preferred option), 33% of surgeons carry out the operation from the left side, 16% choose either position and 6% operate from the right side of the patient. The assistants are positioned on either side of the patient. The number, position and the section of trocars may also differ according to the surgeon's habits and experience and in relationship to the patient's build. Generally the first 10 mm optic trocar is positioned between or over the umbilical area using the open technique. Once the pneumoperitoneum has been insufflated (alternatively the Verres needle can be used) the whole of the abdominal cavity can be explored using a 30° optic.

The other trocars (usually three) are positioned visually. One 5 mm trocar is positioned in the epigastric site to lift the liver and if necessary the gall bladder. The other two trocars are usually positioned in the left abdominal quadrant, on the mid-clavicular line above the umbilical transverse line and on the right side in a position which is diametrically opposite on the projection of the abdominal wall of the transpyloric region. There are other variants in the positioning of the trocars, but the one described seems to best satisfy the requirements of ergonomics and *triangulation* between optics and trocars which are responsible for the uneventful outcome of the laparoscopy.

It is usually easy to identify PPU, even if the missed localization is one of the most frequent reasons for conversion. In the event that the perforation is situated in a *difficult* site (lateral wall of the descending duodenum, posterior gastric wall), some other maneuvers need to be performed, i.e. the mobilization of the duodenum or the section of the gastrocolic ligament in order to reach the retro cavity of the greater omentum.

2.3.5 Closure of the Perforation

The closure of the perforation is probably the most demanding moment of the entire operation and, together with the subsequent extensive washing of the abdominal cavity, is responsible for the longer operating times for the laparoscopy than for the traditional technique. The choice of method of closure depends on the characteristics of the lesion. If the margins are infiltrated, friable and consequently not mobile, the repair should be carried out by positioning an omental patch. For easily joined margins without any tension, a simple suture is sufficient with a possible omental flap. In the latter 2 or 3 sutures are suggested to close the lesion to which in the second moment an omental patch is secured.

As shown in the review by Bertleff [13], ulcer closure is mainly carried out in 66% of cases using the omental patch, less frequently (24%) with the mixed technique (patch + direct suturing) and a small part (10%) with simple direct suturing. The latter is generally used with the intracorporeal techniques (64%), extra-corporeal techniques being used less (14%) or mixed (14%).

The need to principally perform omental patch repair has been emphasized in several studies, in order to reduce the risk of suture line rupture or the enlarging of the lesion (this is possible especially in the case of the ulcer with edematous and friable margins) [9, 13, 41]. Schein [15] even went so far as to state that if omental patch repair is impossible, then gastric resection is required. Walsh et al. [42] have proposed that when on laparoscopic exploration the perforation has been plugged, to leave the omentum in situ and only perform a simple cleaning of the abdominal cavity. As an alternative to classical suturing, several changes have been proposed to simplify the method: *single-stitch laparoscopic repair* [10]; use of a clip to tighten the suture (avoiding a knot in the suture) [43, 44]; using an automated stapler [45] (*stapled omental patch repair*) [46]; reverting to laparoscopic-endoscopic (*gastroscopy-aided repair*) [47].

In order to make the repair of PPU less complex and consequently reducing operating time, the so-called *sutureless* technique has been proposed, which avoids suturing of the perforation (particularly where the margins are friable and edematous). The lesion may be repaired by means of an omental flap placed in situ using fibrin glue (as described by Mouret in the first case of laparoscopy repair in 1990), or by using a plug shaped to the size of the perforation [11, 48, 49]. As demonstrated experimentally by Bertleff et al. [50], this would overcome the problem of the size of the ulcer, which is the drawback of laparoscopic treatment. Nevertheless, there is still an open question whether the reduction of operating time made possible by simpler procedures does not reduce the safety of the laparoscopic technique at the expense of the patient, promoting a greater incidence of postoperative sequelae (in particular leakage) [7, 13].

In this respect, Lee et al. [41] have shown, although without achieving statistical significance, a higher incidence of leakage when *sutureless* techniques are used (only plug with fibrin glue), especially in the case of ulcers more than 5 mm in diameter. These findings were not confirmed by Lau et al. [11] who compared the two techniques (sutures and sutureless) and suggested that the sutureless technique reduces operating times without any difference in terms of morbidity.

2.3.6 Drainage/Lavage

This technique is a fundamental moment during the operation and is performed both in the laparoscopic approach and the open technique. It ensures cleansing of the peritoneal cavity after PPU repair. The withdrawal of intra-abdominal fluids, in particular septic fluids, reduces the occurrence of dangerous postoperative intra-abdominal infections which are often responsible for re-intervention. In this way, compared to the traditional technique laparoscopy offers the advantage of easier access to various intraperitoneal recesses (spaces above and below the liver, left subdiaphragm region, pelvic cavity) without the need to perform extensive and destructive exploratory laparotomies.

There is no agreement in the literature about the amount of saline to use or more importantly whether the lavage is effective in preventing the risk of sepsis (2-6 L of saline are generally recommended, but others recommend using larger quantities, up to 30 L) [7, 13]. However, it is reasonable to perform irrigation only if necessary and, in any case, proportional to the quantity and quality (in particular in the presence of food) of the fluids found in the peritoneal cavity.

There is incomplete agreement on the usage of drainage. It is used only for prophylactic purposes, by the majority of authors [51, 52], positioned in the hepatic region or in the vicinity of the lesion. Only a minority of authors consider it unnecessary [10, 53], seeing it as a possible source of contamination of the peritoneal cavity, as suggested by Petrowsky et al. in a meta-analysis of 2004 [54].

2.3.7 Conversion

In different case studies the percentage of conversion ranges from 0 to 29% [7, 13]. The extreme variability of this figure is probably attributable to the different degree of experience reached by the various surgical teams involved in the studies.

The LAMA randomized, multi-center trial by Bertleff et al. [9] in 2009 shows a conversion rate of about 8%. According to the authors this figure is due to the decent laparoscopic experience acquired by the 9 centers involved in the research (at least 50 previous laparoscopic procedures) and confirms that this type of surgery should only be undertaken by surgeons expert in the field of mini-invasive surgery.

The most common causes for postoperative conversion are due to the size of the perforation (for some authors >6mm [38], for others >10 mm [10]), missed diagnosis, friable margins of the lesion, while localization is predominantly duodenal in 35-65 %, or pyloric in 25-45% contingency [10, 12, 13, 51, 55]), and the severity of peritonitis.

A special condition (which will be discussed below) is suspicion of malignant changes in the ulcer, which is often missed intraoperatively. Regarding this point, performing the biopsy of the ulcer during the same laparoscopic repair of PPU is paramount [56, 57]. For the possible consequences that the conversion involves, it would appear desirable to prevent such a possibility, preferring biopsy rather than resorting to the traditional treatment (undertaking a wide laparotomy with an increase in costs, operating times and morbidity of the abdominal wall). Other risk factors for conversion include the state of shock at the time of hospitalization (risk of conversion up to 50% vs. 8% in patients not in shock) and the time elapsed between the onset of the perforation and diagnosis >24 h (conversion rate up to 33% vs. 0% of patients with no diagnostic delay) [2, 38].

2.3.8 Operating Times

In the meta-analysis by Lau [7] of 2004, operating time was significantly higher for laparoscopy in 5 studies. In a further 5 studies there was no time difference between laparoscopy and open treatment, while only in the RCT by Siu et al. [10] was the operating time lower (42 min for laparoscopy vs. 52.3 min for open treatment). The results obtained in these authors, who are in favor of the laparoscopic approach, is attributed to the particular technique used. This technique uses a single suture point (*single-stitch laparoscopic repair*) for the closure of the PPU and subsequent omental patch [10].

Contrasting results have been reported in the other 2 RCTs by Lau et al. [11] and Bertleff et al. [9], where the results are more favorable for open surgery. The variability of these results can be attributed mainly to the different levels of experience and organization achieved by the surgical teams involved in the study, as well as the technological improvement (in particular the laparoscopic irrigation/drainage system) [7, 10]. These aspects are also emphasized in the systematic review by Lunevicius and Morkevicius [8]. The review states that starting from works published after 2001, the duration of the operation, generally longer in laparoscopy than in open surgery, has undergone a constant and progressive reduction. The authors suggest this is due to technical progress and a better organization acquired over time by the surgical teams. In a retrospective study by the same author in 2005, five independent risk factors responsible for the lengthening of the operating times were identified: These are conversion, a wide perforation, widespread peritonitis, laparoscopy and the patient's state of shock on admission [37].

The LAMA trial of 2009 [9], which shows an average operating time of 50 min for the open technique and 75 min for laparoscopy, justifies such results because of the major technical difficulties with the laparoscopic suturing, especially in the case of an ulcer with friable margins. In this context it is has been highlighted that the use of easier techniques such as *sutureless* repair can help to reduce the operating time, as has already been shown by the 1996 RCT by Lau et al. [11]. In the same trial, another reason responsible for the lengthening of the operation was identified, i.e. the washing procedure and aspiration of peritoneal recesses, due to the decrease of the pneumoperitoneum and the consequent reduction of operating space [9].

2.3.9 Reintervention

The systematic review conducted by Lunevicius and Morkevicius [8] on seven studies revealed no statistically significant difference between the incidence of reoperation between the laparoscopic approach and the open technique, although the incidence is almost double after laparoscopy (5.3% vs. 2.1%). Also in the meta-analysis by Lau [7] the incidence of reoperation is significantly higher after laparoscopy (3.7 %) than after traditional surgery (1.6%). The most frequent complication which requires re operation is suture leakage (7 cases).

2.3.10 Postoperative Pain

The meta-analysis conducted by Lau in 2004 [7] was the first on this topic and included 13 trials (with 2 RCTs [10, 11]) for a total of 658 patients. These patients all underwent laparoscopic repair of a PPU (with the exception of sutureless techniques). One of the parameters for the laparoscopic approach was postoperative pain. Out of 10 studies reviewed, Lau et al. [11] showed a significant reduction in the dose of analgesics. Three other studies [10, 11, 58] where the VAS pain score was being used confirmed that the values are significantly reduced after laparoscopy. Only in the trial by Siu et al. [10] was a statistically significant difference shown, in particular in the first 3 post-op days.

In contrast, in the RCT by Lau the earlier measurements (first 24 h postoperative) can overlap in the two techniques (open and laparoscopic) [11]. Probably in these situations, because the pain is caused mainly by peritoneal inflammation the positive effect is temporarily reduced through reduced damage to the parietal wall by the use of the laparoscopic approach [55]. These results were confirmed in a later LAMA trial [9] and in systematic reviews carried out by Lunevicius and Morkevicius [8] and Sanabria et al. [5, 6].

2.3.11 Complications

In the evaluation of postoperative morbidity, the parameters most frequently taken into consideration are sepsis sequelae (generalized sepsis, infection of the wall, intra-abdominal abscesses, lung infections), complications of the perforated lesion (rupture of suturing, hemorrhage, recurrence of the ulcer), systemic complications (e.g. cardiovascular) or other conditions such as prolonged dynamic ileus.

The first RCT on the use of laparoscopy in PPU by Lau et al. [11] published in 1996 compared the different surgical techniques (open vs. laparoscopy and sutures vs. sutureless repair), pointing out that in terms of mortality and morbidity there were no statistically significant differences between the two methods of mini-invasive and traditional, nor between sutures and sutureless repair techniques.

These results have since been confirmed by other studies, including a further 2 RCTs available on the subject. They reaffirm the excellence of the laparoscopic option in terms of security and feasibility [9, 10]. A more recent meta-analysis by Lau [7] and a systematic review by Lunevicius and Morkevicius [8] reported significantly lower mortality rates (even if not statistically significant) compared to those recorded after open treatment (respectively 4.8% vs. 10.2% in Lau and 3.9% vs. 11.0% in Lunevicius). The patients who are most at risk are those in poor general health with at least one of the Boey risk factors present. In the two studies [7, 8] the overall incidence of complications can also be overlapped for laparoscopy and open surgery.

In a more detailed analysis of the individual complications, the authors of both studies show no statistically significant difference between the two types of intervention in the incidence of intra-abdominal abscesses (which are higher after laparoscopic treatment), postoperative ileus (more frequent after open treatment) or lung infections (considered the most frequent cause of morbidity).

However, the rate of abdominal wall sepsis is greatly reduced after laparoscopy than after traditional surgery (respectively 2.1 vs. 6.9; p=0.036 in Lau and 2.5% vs. 6.9%; p=0.006 in Lunevicius and Morkevicius [8], with a consequent reduction in the incidence of an incisional hernia. In contrast, a higher incidence of suture leakage after laparoscopy has been demonstrated: 3.9% vs. 2.6% of traditional surgery in Lau [7] and 6.9% vs. 1.3% in Lunevicius and Morkevicius [8]. This figure is not statistically significant, particularly when separately examining the results of the 2 RCTs [10, 11] included in reviews. In particular, Siu et al. [52] stress the incidence of leakage in relation to the size of the ulcer: low incidence (< 2%) if the diameter of the lesion is <10 mm.

Lee et al. [41] has identified APACHE II (>5 points) and ulcer diameter (>10mm) as factors independent of the risk of post-op leakage in patients undergoing sutureless (plug with fibrin glue) laparoscopic repair of PPU. The importance of the experience gained by the surgeon in the field of mini-invasive surgery was emphasized in this case. In a study by Lunevicius and Morkevicius [37], all cases of suture leakage are reported when the intervention is carried out by surgeons with limited learning curves (less than 10 laparoscopic suturings). The most recent studies, as the 2010 review by Bertleff and Lange shows [13], confirm the previous data concerning equivalence of the rate of complications between the two methods and a lower incidence of mortality after laparoscopy: 14.3% and 3.6% vs. 28.3% and 6.4%, respectively after laparoscopy and open surgery. The review by Sanabria et al. (recently updated to 2010) [5, 6] is also an indication of the trend towards a decrease in some complications such as abdominal infections, post-op ileus, pulmonary infections, as well as the mortality rate, after laparoscopic surgery, although none of these results are statistically significant.

In contrast, although not statistically significant, the incidence of intra-abdominal abscesses and reintervention in comparison with traditional surgery has increased. Lastly, no conclusion has been reached with regard to other complications, such as the incidence of a ruptured suture line or the risk of incisional hernia.

2.3.12 Hospitalization

All studies have reported favorable results for laparoscopy in terms of post-op hospitalization period or at any rate no worse than those after traditional surgery [7-11]. This is highlighted in the 3 most important systematic reviews by Lau (3 studies out of 13 favorable and 10 with comparable results) [7], Lunevicius and Morkevicius (4 studies out 15 favorable and 11 comparable) [8] and Sanabria et al. (1 study out of 3 favorable and 2 comparable) [6]. Siu et al. [10], while highlighting that no significant differences between the two methods are evident (the timing of the removal of the nasogastric tube, suspension of parenteral therapy and the resumption of oral diet), does report a reduction in hospitalization (6 vs 7 days; $p= <0.001$) and consequently an earlier return to normal activities (10.4 vs. 26.1 days, $p=0.001$) by the patient treated laparoscopically than those treated traditionally. The LAMA multicenter trial conducted by Bertleff et al. [9] reports a reduced hospital stay after laparoscopy: 6.5 vs. 8.0; $p=0.235$. In confirming the overlapping of the two methods in terms of postoperative hospitalization and resumption of normal activities on the part of the patient, Lunevicius and Morkevicius [12] stress that these aspects are also linked to factors outside the medical field, pertaining to the cultural habits of the patient and the different health policies followed by the various surgical centers involved. In addition, the benefits do not appear as evident as in the treatment of other diseases (e.g. VL cholecystectomy), because the patients treated have peritonitis and are often elderly, so they require a longer hospital stay.

2.3.13 Definitive Surgery of the Peptic Ulcer

The introduction of drugs able to control hyperacidity and the radical treatment of HP made possible by antibiotics have led on the one hand to a reduced need for *acid-reductive* surgery and on the other hand a reduction of ulcerative recurrences (and so the need for re-intervention surgery) [43, 44, 59]. Nevertheless, up to 35% of patients who have undergone PPU may require definitive surgical treatment, which may be conducted laparoscopically in relation to the degree of the surgeon's skill, considering also the overlapping results which compare the open technique: recurrence of the ulcer from 4 to 11%; post-op complications 1–2% [12, 13].

The indications for *acid-reductive* surgery, (vagotomy, gastric resection) should be reserved for non-responders (ineffectiveness of the drug, the inability of the patient to comply with treatment over the medium- to long-term, costs of medicines, relapse after discontinuation of therapy), in the presence of PPU complicated by hemorrhage, or in the presence of complications of chronic PPU like stenosis. The possibility of a perforated gastric cancer is a particular condition, which we will discuss in the next section [12].

2.3.14 Perforated Gastric Cancer

Due to various diagnostic and therapeutic problems we refer to this situation separately. Gastric cancer is diagnosed with difficulty (only about 30% of cases) and often during the operation it is indistinguishable from a benign ulcer unless a biopsy of the ulcerative lesion is performed. This is recommended as routine by some authors for all gastric perforations [56, 57]. In addition, no definitive conclusions can be reached in terms of treatment strategy. The perforation of a gastric cancer is rare (1% of gastric cancers and about 10–16% of gastric perforation should be suspected in patients over 65) [56]. The studies available consist of a limited number of cases which only refer to open treatment and significant results on the treatment of this disease in emergency surgery cannot be obtained.

From the initial experiences by Rubh Aird [60] in 1935 until the early 1980s the most frequent type of intervention was the simple closure of the ulcer, possibly associated with omental patch repair. Despite the associated high mortality, the intervention was justified by the conviction that the spreading of tumor cells secondary to the perforation was the expression of advanced disease with serosal invasion (55-82%) and lymph node metastases (57-67%) [60].

Several studies have shown that a perforation can complicate the gastric cancer, even in the early stages [56]. In addition, recent data suggest that a perforation and consequent peritoneal spread of tumor cells does not necessarily affect survival in patients undergoing resective surgery. This has been shown by several studies where the survival at 5 years in patients with a perforated gastric cancer is the same as a non-complicated gastric cancer [57, 60-65]. A multivariate analysis has shown that the degree of lymph node invasion is the only factor related to long-term survival of patients with perforated gastric cancer [66]. All this has meant that in recent years, even in the presence of a perforated gastric cancer, resective surgery has gained ground, with increasingly encouraging results on selected patients, in terms of surgical mortality and long-term survival rates [61, 62, 66].

In 2002 Lehnert et al. [62] proposed a two-phase operation: the first, a simple repair of the perforation; the second a radical gastrectomy. This approach would fully meet two fundamental requirements: avoid major surgical procedures in a frail patient because of peritonitis and cancer; improve the patient's clinical condition and after appropriate cancer staging perform the correct oncologic procedure.

2.3.15 Nonoperative Management

Studies by Taylor [67] in the first half of the 20th century have shown that at least half of the patients with PPU are buffered by the positive effects of the adjacent organs, in particular by the greater omentum. This has tended to suggest that nonoperative management (NOM) is a possible valid alternative to surgery for PPU in selected cases. In the past, high rates of morbidity and mortality in PPU surgery have in certain situations convinced several surgeons to give priority to conservative treatment.

Today, thanks to the latest progress made by laparoscopic surgery, the indication for this option has been greatly reduced. It has been shown that the mortality rates of NOM have remained stable (from 5.2% of the initial experience by Taylor in 1957, to rates ranging between 0 and 8% in recent publications), while the percentage of procedure failure with possible septic shock, multiple organ failure or development of intra-abdominal abscesses is significant (between 13 and 46% in the literature) and these patients are in their turn exposed to the risk of delayed surgical treatment, with its associated increased mortality (3-50% of cases) [68, 69].

Compared to the initial experience by Taylor, who had restricted NOM to patients in good health, other authors have reported good results in a selected category of patients. According to Croft [68] and Marshall [69] possible indications for NOM are the onset of symptoms of less than 24 hours, the presence of slight abdominal pain with minimal peritoneal irritation, hemodynamic stability with no signs of sepsis in patients under the age of 70 years. The CT scan of the abdomen or a gastroduodenography with a water soluble contrast medium is mandatory to quantify the presence and extent of loss of intraperitoneal gastroduodenal liquid. Patients with minimal perforations and no leakage are nominated for NOM. In contrast, patients with unstable hemodynamics, symptom duration of more than 24 hours, severe peritonitis, diffuse sepsis and age >70 years should undergo emergent surgery [68, 69].

The positioning of a nasogastric tube, instauration of parenteral therapy, administration of proton pump inhibitor (PPI) therapy together with an adequate antibiotic therapy (the so-called *Taylor method*), should lead to a rapid improvement (within 12 hours) in the patient's clinical condition. NOM should be interrupted opting for surgical treatment if no significant improvement has been seen during this time. The RCT by Croft, where conservative and surgical treatment are compared, shows similar results in terms of morbidity and mortality. Two aspects are different: (1) a longer hospital stay in the group who underwent NOM; (2) the rates of failure of conservative treatment significantly higher in patients >70 years compared to <40 years (respectively by 67% and 0%) [68].

Bucher et al. [70] performed NOM on inoperable patients because of their poor clinical condition. The authors pointed out that the eradication of HP and especially the introduction of PPI drugs can positively influence the results of conservative treatment (mortality by 64% in the group of patients with H_2-blockers, compared to 11% of the patients in therapy with PPI). On the other hand, shock is the greatest predictive criterion for the failure of NOM (while no influence would be given to the advanced age of the patient), so patients who are hemodynamically unstable should be candidates for surgery without delay [70]. Lagoo et al. [2] in virtue of their progress in the field of laparoscopy, restrict the use of NOM to patients with a buffered perforation who are unable to undergo surgery because of their poor general health and terminal septic shock.

2.4 Conclusions

In the light of the most recent studies, the laparoscopic approach can be seen as a possible alternative to traditional treatment in the correction of the PPU, and a feasible and sufficiently secure method if conducted by expert hands in properly selected patients.

The results of the most recent literature confirm that, compared to traditional surgery, the use of laparoscopy decreases postoperative pain and several complications (infection of the abdominal wall, prolonged post-op ileus, pulmonary infections and mortality rates). None of these results is statistically significant. In contrast, an increase (also not statistically significant) in the incidence of intra-abdominal abscesses and recurrences caused mostly by suture leakage has also been reported. The operating times for laparoscopy are higher, despite the experience obtained over the last decade which has led to its progressive reduction. This is probably due to the greater experience gained by the surgeon as a result of technical progress and organization acquired over time by the surgical teams.

It is widely believed that such data, far from being able to be considered as definitive, deserve further evaluation, and, especially, require wider and more numerous trials of quality (randomized prospective studies). The best and most recent systematic review by Sanabria et al., updated to 2010 [6], involves only 3 RCTs [9-11] (evaluated of acceptable quality), for a small diversified sample of just 315 patients.

The best definition of prognostic criteria able to identify patients at higher risk for laparoscopic surgery as well as the determination of predictive factors of laparoscopy-to-open conversion are some of the priority objectives to be pursued. Currently the most important reference criteria are a high Boey score and patient age >70 years. In the presence of these conditions, the laparoscopic option should be contraindicated due to the high risk of morbidity and mortality. However, given the limited experience in the use of laparoscopy in these high-risk patients, it is not possible to make definitive judgments on the selection of patients who could undergo mini-invasive treatment of PPU and, in particular, on those patients where the use of laparoscopy should be categorically ruled out. There is a certain degree of variability in the techniques used in laparoscopy for the repair of the PPU. The ideal technique should meet some fundamental requirements, such as the relative ease of implementation with reduction of operating time (and consequently the risk for the patient and the costs of the procedure) and reliability, in terms of reduced morbidity (in particular for a reduction in the risk of leakage). The criterion of choice for the closure method depends fundamentally on the characteristics of the lesion. If lesion margins can be easily joined without tension, a simple suture is sufficient with possible omental patch. If the margins are edematous or not mobile, the repair must be performed by affixing an omental patch. The use of the *sutureless* technique aims to facilitate the closure of the PPU, avoiding the use of sutures and consequently reducing the operating time. However, further studies are needed to verify whether these benefits are not offset by reduced safety for the patient in terms of increased morbidity (suture leakage).

The degree of experience achieved by surgical teams who use the laparoscopic technique to treat PPU is one of the most relevant prognostic factors for the purposes of the end result, even if to date this is extremely difficult to determine. Some data, such as the progressive reduction of operating times and conversion rates, together with the increase in the number of patients undergoing laparoscopy for PPU, can be considered as indicative parameters for the purposes of assessing the level reached by the surgeons in this type of surgery. However, further studies are needed in the future to better define this aspect, with particular reference to laparoscopic learning curves, necessary to envision in relative safety this type of disease.

No reference is present in the literature about the costs of laparoscopic surgery. However, it seems reasonable to assume that the reduction in operating time, linked to the greater experience and improved organizational capacity of the surgical teams, as well as the progress in the field of technology, can in the near future lead to a reduction in operating costs closely related to the operation. On the other hand, an overall estimate of the costs, including post-op hospital stay and return to work or daily activities appears to be more complex. The progressive increase in the elderly suffering from PPU, often in the presence of a clinical picture of peritonitis, may in fact represent an obstacle to a more rapid discharge and consequently to an immediate resumption of normal activities on the part of the patient.

References

1. Lui FY, Davis KA (2010) Gastroduodenal perforation: maximal or minimal intervention? Scand J Surg 99:73-77
2. Lagoo S, McMahon RL, Kalkharu M et al (2002) The sixth decision regarding perforated duodenal ulcer. JSLS 6:359-368
3. Mouret J, Francois Y, Vignal J et al (1990) Laparoscopic treatment of perforated duodenal ulcer. Br J Surg 77:1006
4. Nathanson LK, Easter DW, Cuschieri A (1990) Laparoscopic repair peritoneal toilette of perforated duodenal ulcer. Surg Endosc 4:232-233
5. Sanabria AE, Morales CH, Villegas MI (2005) Laparoscopic repair for perforated peptic ulcer disease. Cochrane Database Syst Rev 4:CD004778
6. Sanabria AE, Morales CH, Villegas MI (2005) Laparoscopic repair for perforated peptic ulcer disease. The Cochrane Library 4[Last assessed as up-to-date: March 9 2010] DOI: 10.1002/14651858.CD004778.pub2
7. Lau H (2004) Laparoscopic repair of perforated peptic ulcer. A meta-analysis. Surg Endosc 18:1013-1021
8. Lunevicius R, Morkevicius M (2005) Systemic review comparing laparoscopic and open repair for perforated peptic ulcer. Br J Surg 92:1195-1207

9. Bertleff M, Halm JA, Bemelman WA et al (2009) Randomized clinical trial of laparoscopic versus open repair of the perforated peptic ulcer: the LAMA trial. World J Surg 33:1368-1373
10. Siu WT, Leong HT, Law BKB et al (2002) Laparoscopic repair for perforated peptic ulcer: a randomized controlled trial. Ann Surg 235:313-319
11. Lau WY, Leung KL, Kwong KH et al (1996) A randomized study comparing laparoscopic versus open repair of perforated peptic ulcer using suture or sutureless technique. Ann Surg 224:131-138
12. Lunevicius R, Morkevicius M (2005) Management strategies, early results, benefits and risk factors of laparoscopic repair of perforated peptic ulcer. World J Surg 29:1299-1310
13. Bertleff M, Lange JF (2010) Laparoscopic correction of perforated peptic ulcer: first choice? A review of literature. Surg Endosc 24:1231-1239
14. Kakhry S, Watts D, Daley B et al (2001) Current diagnostic approach lack sensitivity in the diagnosis of perforating blunt small bowel injury (SBI): findings from a large multi-institutional trial. J Trauma 51:1232
15. Schein M (2010) Perforated peptic ulcer. In: Schein M, Rogers PN, Assalia A (eds) Schein's common sense emergency abdominal surgery, Springer, Berlin Heidelberg, pp 157-166
16. Miller RE, Nelson SW (1971) The roentgenologic demonstration of tiny amounts of free intarperitoneal gas: experimental and clinical studies. AJR Am J Roentgenol 112:574-585
17. Chen SC, Wang HP, Chen WJ (2002) Selective use of ultrasonography for the detection of pneumoperitoneum. Acad Emerg Med 9:643-645
18. Phatak Mg, Frank SJ, Ellis JJ (1984) Computed tomography of bowel perforation. Gastrointest Radiol 9:133-135
19. Cho KC, Baker SR (1994) Extraluminal air: diagnosis and significance. Radiol Clin North Am 32:829-844
20. Stapakis JC, Thickman D (1992) Diagnosis of pneumoperitoneum: abdominal CT vs upright chest film. J Comput Assist Tomogr 16:713-716
21. Earls JP, Dachaman AH, Colon E et al (1993) Prevalence and duration of postoperative pneumoperitoneum: sensitivity of CT vs left lateral decubits radiography. AJR 161:781-785
22. Chen CH, Huang HS, Yang CC, Yeh YH (2001) Features of perforated peptic ulcers in conventional computed tomography. Hepatogastroenterology 48:1393-1396
23. Fultz PJ, Skucas J, Weiss SL (1992) CT in upper gastrointestinal tract perforations secondary to peptic ulcer disease. Gastrointest Radiol 17:5-8
24. Hainaux B, Agneessen E, Bertinotti R et al (2006) Accuracy of MDCT in predicting site of gastrointestinal tract perforation. AJR 187:1179-1183
25. Imuta M, Awai K, Nakayama Y et al (2004) Multidetector CT findings suggesting a perforation site in the gastrointestinal tract: analysis in surgical confirmed 155 patients. Imaging 28:334-339
26. Rice RP, Thompson WM, Gedgaudas RK (1982) The diagnosis and significance of extraluminal gas in the abdomen. Radiol Clin North Am 20:819-837
27. Cho HS, Yoon SE, Park SH et al (2009) Distinction between upper and lower gastrointestinal perforation. Usefulness of the periportal free air sign on computed tomography. Eur J Radiol 69:108-113
28. Ghekiere O, Lesnik A, Hoa D et al (2007) Value of computed tomography in the diagnosis of the cause of non traumatic gastrointestinal tract perforation. J Comput Assist Tomogr 31:169-176
29. Maniatis V, Chryssikopoulos H, Roussakis A et al (2000) Perforation of the alimentary tract: evaluation with computed tomography. Abdom Imaging 25:373-379
30. Brenner DJ, Hall EJ (2007) Computed tomography: an increasing source of radiation exposure. N Engl J Med 357:2277-2284
31. Moriwaki Y, Sugiyama M, Toyoda H (2009) Ultrasonography for the diagnosis of the intraperitoneal free air on chest-abdominal-pelvic blunt trauma and critical acute abdominal pain. Arch Surg 144:137-141
32. Singh JP, Steward MJ, Booth TG et al (2010) Evolution of imaging for abdominal perforation. Ann R Coll Surg Engl 92:182-188

33. Agresta F, Mazzarolo G, Ciardo LF, Bedin N (2005) The laparoscopic approach in abdominal emergiencies: has the attitude changed? A single-center review of a 15 year experience. Surg Endosc 22:1255-1262
34. Bhogal R, Athwal R, Durkin D et al (2008) Comparison between open and laparoscopic repair of perforated peptic ulcer disease. Worl J Surg 32:2371-2374
35. Ates M, Coban S, Sevil S, Terzi A (2008) The efficacy of laparoscopic surgery in patients with peritonitis. Surg Laparosc Endosc Percutan Tech 18:453-456
36. Boey J, Wong J (1987) Perforated duodenal ulcers. World J Surg 11:319-324
37. Lunevicius R, Morkevicius M (2005) Comparison of laparoscopic versus open repair for perforated duodenal ulcers. Surg Endosc 19:1565-1571
38. Katkhouda N, Mavor E, Mason RJ et al (1999) Laparoscopic repair of perforated duodenal ulcers: outcome and efficacy in 30 consecutive patients. Arch Surg 134:845-850
39. Robertson GS, Wemyss-Holden SA, Maddern GJ (2000) Laparoscopic repair of perforated duodenal ulcers. The role of laparoscopy in generalized peritonitis. Ann R Coll Surg Engl 82:6-10
40. Vaidya BB, Garg CP, Shah JP (2009) Laparoscopic repair of perforated peptic ulcer with delayed presentation. J Laparosc Adv Surg Tech 19:153-156
41. Lee FY, Leung KL, Lai BS et al (2001) Predicting mortality and morbility of patients operated on for perforated peptic ulcers. Arch Surg 136:90-94
42. Walsh CJ, Khoo DE, Motson RW (1993) Laparoscopic repair of perforated peptic ulcer. Br J Surg 80:127
43. Wemyss-Holden S, White SA, Robertson G, Lloyd D (2002) Color coding of sutures in laparoscopic perforated duodenal ulcer: a new concept. Surg Laparosc Endosc Percutan Tech 12:177-179
44. Matsuda M, Nishiyama M, Hanai T et al (1995) Laparoscopic omental patch repair for perforated peptic ulcer. Ann Surg 221:236-240
45. Guglielminotti P, Bini R, Fontana D, Leli R (2009) Laparoscopic repair for perforated peptic ulcers with U-CLIP. World J Emerg Surg 4:28
46. Darzi A, Chesire NJ, Somers SS (1993) Laparoscopic omental patch repair with an automated stapler. Br J Surg 80:1552
47. Costalat G, Alquier Y (1995) Combined laparoscopic and endoscopic treatment of perforated gastroduodenal ulcers using the ligamentum teres hepatis. Surg Endosc 9:677-679
48. Tate JJT, Dawson JW, Lau WY et al (1993) Sutureless laparoscopic treatment of perforated duodenal ulcer. Br J Surg 80:235
49. Tate JJT, Dawson JW, Lau WY et al (1993) Sutureless laparoscopic treatment of perforated duodenal ulcer. Br J Surg 80:235
50. Bertleff M, Stegmann T, Liem R et al (2009) Comparison of closure of gastric perforation ulcers with biodegradable lactide-glycolide-caprolactone or omental patches. JSLS 13:550-554
51. Druart ML, Van Hee R, Etienne J et al (1997) Laparoscopic repair of perforated duodenal ulcer. A prospective multicenter clinical trial. Surg Endosc 11:1017-1020
52. Siu WT, Chau CH, Law BKB et al (2004) Routine use of laparoscopic repair for perforated peptic ulcer. Br J Surg 91:481-484
53. Cellan-Jones CJ (1929) A rapid method of treatment in perforated duodenal ulcer. BMJ 1:1076-1077.
54. Petrowsky H, Demartines N, Rousson V, Clavien PA (2004) Evidence-based value of prophylactic drainage in gastrointestinal surgery. A systematic review and meta-analyses. Ann Surg 240:1074-1085
55. Naegaard JM, Edwin B, Reiertsen O et al (1999) Laparoscopic and open operation in patients with perforated peptic ulcer. Eur J Surg 165:209-214
56. Adachi Y, Mori M, Maehara Y et al (1997) Surgical results of perforated gastric carcinoma: an analysis of 155 Japanese patients. Am J Gastroenterol 92:516-548
57. Roviello F, Rossi S, Marrelli D et al (2006) Perforated gastric carcinoma: a report of 10 cases and review of the literature. World J Surg Oncol 4:19
58. Miserez M, Eypasch E, Spangenberger W et al (1996) Laparoscopic and conventional closure of perforated peptic ulcer: a comparison. Surg Endosc 10:831-836

59. Pappas TN, Lagoo SA (2002) Laparoscopic repair for perforated peptic ulcer. Ann Surg 235:320-321
60. Aird I (1935) Perforation of carcinoma of the stomach into the general peritoneal cavity. Br J Surg 22:545-554
61. Lee HJ, Park DJ, Yang HK et al (2006) Outcome after emergency surgery in gastric cancer patients with free perforation or severe bleeding. Dig Surg 23:217-223
62. Lehnert T, Buhl K, Dueck M et al (2000) Two-staged radical gastrectomy for perforated gastric cancer. Eur J Surg Oncol 26:780-784
63. Kitakado Y, Tanigawa N, Muraoka R (1997) A case report perforated early gastric cancer. Nippon Geka Hokan 66:86-90
64. Kasakura Y, Ajai JA, Mochizuki F et al (2002) Outcomes after emergency surgery for gastric perforation or severe bleeding in patients with gastric cancer. J Surg Oncol 7:219-224
65. So JB, Yam A, Cheah WK et al (2000) Risk factors related to operative mortality and morbility in patients undergoing emergency gastrectomy. Br J Surg 87:1702-1707
66. Gertsch P, Yip SK, Chow LW, Launder IJ (1995) Free perforation of gastric carcinoma. Arch Surg 130: 177-181
67. Taylor H (1957) The non-surgical treatment of perforated peptic ulcer. Gastroenterology 33:353-368
68. Croft TJ, Kenneth GM, Park MB (1989) A randomized trial of non operative treatment for perforated duodenal ulcer. N Engl J Med 320:970-973
69. Marshall C, Ramanswamy P, Bergin FG et al (1999) Evaluation of a protocol for the nonoperative management of perforated peptic ulcer. Br J Surg 86:131-134
70. Bucher P, Oulbaci W, Morel P et al (2007) Results of conservative treatment for perforated gastroduodenal ulcer in patients not eligible for surgical repair. Swiss Med WKLY 137:337-340
71. Notashi AY, Salimi J, Rahimian H et al (2005) Evaluation of Mannheim Peritonitis Index and multiple failure score in patients with peritonitis. Ind J Gastroenterol 24:197-200

Suggested Readings

Sauerland S, Agresta F, Bergamaschi R, Borzellino G, Budzynski A, Champault G, Fingerhut A, Isla A, Johansson M, Lundorff P (2006) Laparoscopy for abdominal emergencies. Evidence-based guidelines of the European Association for Endoscopic Surgery. Surg Endosc 20:14–29

Agresta F, Ansaloni L, Baiocchi L, Bergamini C, Campanile FB, Carlucci M, Cocorullo G, Corradi A, Franzato B, Lupo M, Mandalà V, Mirabella A, Pernazza G, Piccoli M, Staudacher C, Vettoretto N, Zago M, Lettieri E, Levati A, Pietrini D, Scaglione M, De Masi S, De Placido G, Francucci M, Rasi M, Scaramuzza G, Del Favero AL (2011) Consensus Development Conference of the Società Italiana Chirurgia Endoscopica e nuove tecnologie (SICE); Associazione Chirurghi Ospedalieri Italiani (ACOI); Società Italiana di Chirurgia (SIC); Società Italiana Chirurgia d'Urgenza e Trauma (SICUT), Società Italiana Chirurghi dell'Ospedalità Privata (SICOP) and the European Association for Endoscopic Surgery (EAES). In press

Acute Cholecystitis

3

Fabio Cesare Campanile, Paolo Colobraro, Nicola Foti,
Massimo Lupo and Vincenzo Mandalà

3.1 Introduction

Acute cholecystitis is an acute inflammatory disease of the gallbladder, often due to gallstones. Between 3% and 10% of all patients with abdominal pain have acute cholecystitis [1] (Fig. 3.1).

Cholelithiasis accounts for more than 90% of causes of acute cholecystitis [2, 3], the remaining 10% (acalculous cholecystitis) are generally associated with trauma, burns, recent surgery, multisystem organ failure, parenteral nutrition, AIDS or ischemia [4-6].

About 10-15% of the adult population of Western countries have gallstones [7-10]. In the USA a prevalence of 20 million people with cholelithiasis is estimated [11]. Each year 1-4% become symptomatic [12] and cholecystectomy is the most common operation performed on the digestive system. About 700,000 cholecystectomies are performed annually in the US [13]. In Italy about 102,000 cholecystectomies were performed in 2009 [14]. Between 70 and 90 per cent of all cholecystectomies are operated on laparoscopically [14, 16] and about 10-30% for acute cholecystitis [16, 17].

The laparoscopic approach was initially considered to be contraindicated for acute cholecystitis was but it adopted later, as experience increased, gradually overtaking open cholecystectomy as the preferred procedure even in an acute setting.

The severity of the disease may range from a mild, self-limited illness to a severe, potentially life-threatening illness.

Between 50 and 70% of the cases of acute cholecystitis occur in aged patients [18] and a steady increase in life expectancy during the past years will

F.C. Campanile (✉)
General Surgery, Andosilla Hospital,
Civita Castellana (VT), Italy

V. Mandalà, *The Role of Laparoscopy in Emergency Abdominal Surgery*,

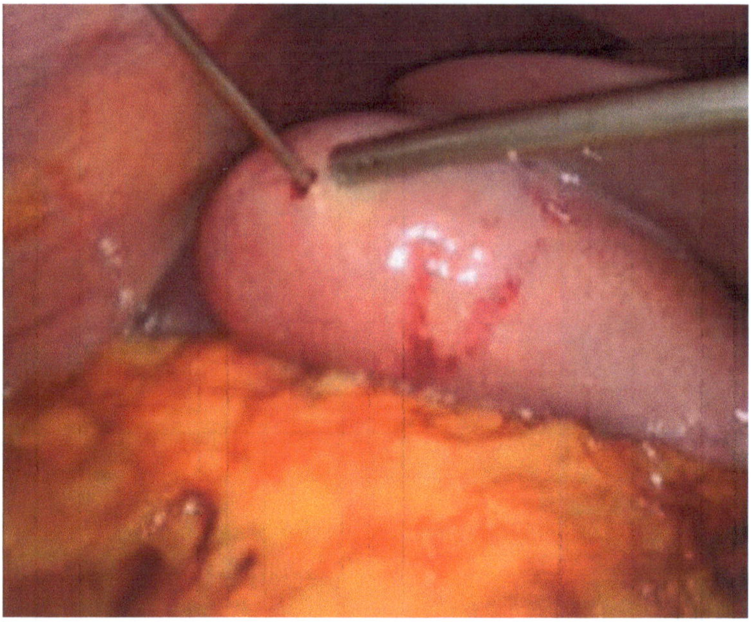

Fig. 3.1 Acute purulent cholecystitis. Previous aspiration of the gallbladder

make the problem even more relevant in the future. High prevalence of co-morbidities in the elderly, as well as increased incidence of complications, sepsis and severe forms of cholecystitis in this particular population often causes a serious surgical emergency.

Several international guidelines have addressed the issue of diagnosis and treatment of acute cholecystitis [19-23].

3.2 Diagnosis and Staging

Diagnosis of acute cholecystitis relies on a combination of local clinical signs, systemic signs of inflammation and imaging findings. Very similar sets of criteria able to achieve almost 100% specificity have been suggested in the European Association of Endoscopic Surgery (EAES) guidelines of 2006 [19] and in the Tokyo Consensus Meeting Guidelines [20] and both can be used in clinical practice.

In the EAES guidelines a set of criteria validated by a systematic review (EL1a) has been adopted: (a) acute right upper quadrant tenderness for more than 6 h and ultrasound evidence of acute cholecystitis (the presence of gallstones with a thickened and edematous gallbladder wall, positive Murphy's sign on ultrasound examination, and pericholecystic fluid collections) or (b) acute right upper quadrant tenderness for more than 6 h, an ultrasound image

Table 3.1 Diagnostic criteria for acute cholecystitis

(A)	Local signs of inflammation
	Murphy's sign
	RUQ mass/pain/tenderness
(B)	Systemic signs of inflammation
	Fever
	Elevated CRP (>3mg/dL)(EL 1b) [25]
	Elevated WBC count
(C)	Imaging findings
	Imaging findings characteristic of acute cholecystitis
	Definitive diagnosis
(1)	One item in A and one item in B are positive
(2)	C confirms the diagnosis when acute cholecystitis is suspected clinically. NB: acute hepatitis, other acute abdominal diseases and chronic cholecystitis should be ruled out

Table 3.2 Imaging findings of acute cholecystitis

Ultrasonography findings (EL 4)
Sonographic Murphy sign (tenderness elicited by pressing the gallbladder with the ultrasound probe)
Thickened gallbladder wall (>4 mm; if the patient does not have chronic liver disease and/or ascites or right heart failure)
Enlarged gallbladder (long axis diameter >8 cm, short axis diameter >4 cm)
Incarcerated gallstone, debris echo, pericholecystic fluid collection
Sonolucent layer in the gallbladder wall, striated intramural lucencies, and Doppler signals
Magnetic resonance imaging findings (EL 1b-4)
Pericholecystic high signal
Enlarged gallbladder
Thickened gallbladder wall
Computed tomography findings (EL 3b)
Thickened gallbladder wall
Pericholecystic fluid collection
Enlarged gallbladder
Linear high-density areas in the pericholecystic fat tissue

showing the presence of gallstones, and one or more of the following: temperature above 38° C, leukocytosis [24], and/or C-reactive protein level greater than 10 mg/L.

The criteria of the Tokyo Consensus Meeting Guidelines are summarized in Tables 3.1 and 3.2.

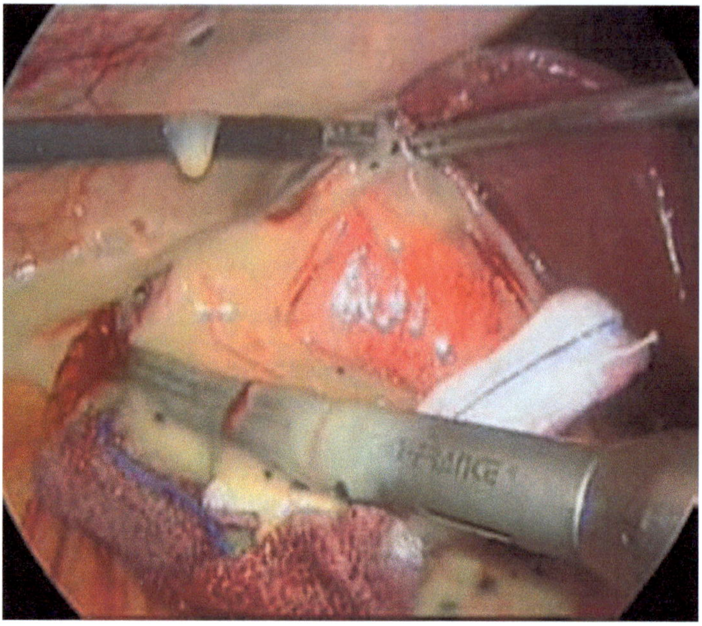

Fig. 3.2 Despite the spillage of pus, the rapid aspiration and sequential washing avoided postoperative abscesses in the abdominal cavity and abdominal wall. Observation V. Mandalà

Ultrasound (US) is the preferred initial modality in the investigation of right upper quadrant pain [26]. It is more sensitive than computed tomography (CT) in the diagnosis of acute cholecystitis. Magnetic resonance imaging (MRI) is playing an increasing role in the evaluation of acute abdominal pain, particularly for pediatric and pregnant patients. MRI has sensitivity of 95% and specificity of 69% for the detection of acute cholecystitis [27]. Magnetic resonance cholangiopancreatography (MRCP) is more sensitive than US (sensitivity 100%, specificity 93% and accuracy 97% vs. sensitivity 62%, specificity 100% and accuracy 77%) in the depiction of cystic duct and gallbladder neck calculi and the evaluation of cystic duct obstruction [28].

A prospective randomized study showed that the association of elevated C-reactive protein (3mg/dL or more) and US findings suggesting acute cholecystitis has a sensitivity of 97%, specificity of 76%, and positive predictive value of 95% [25].

Most patients with acute cholecystitis present with a mild form of the disease, although about one third of them progress to a possibly life threatening severe form [29]. The worsening of the inflammatory process and bacterial colonization of the gallbladder wall can cause the formation of necrosis or purulent collections and, through the action of mediators, can impair the function of distant organs, up to sepsis and death. Several factors have been associated with progression to a severe form of cholecystitis (empyematous, gangrenous or perforated): age, male gender, cardiovascular disease and diabetes (Fig. 3.2).

Most authors stage the severity of the disease on the basis of local findings only (*severe cholecystitis* = empyematous, gangrenous or perforated) [29]); recent guidelines (Tokyo Guidelines, 2007) [20]) include criteria concerning organ dysfunction and suggest a staging system based on three grades: *mild* acute cholecystitis (Grade I) is an acute form in a healthy patient with no organ dysfunction and only mild inflammatory local changes; the more severe forms are further divided in two grades, based on the presence or absence of organ dysfunction: *moderate* acute cholecystitis (Grade II) if marked local inflammation (biliary peritonitis, pericholecystic abscess, hepatic abscess, gangrenous cholecystitis, emphysematous cholecystitis) is demonstrated, or if preoperative findings suggest marked inflammation (WBC count >18 000/mm^3, palpable tender mass in the right upper quadrant or duration of symptoms >72 h); *severe* acute cholecystitis (Grade III) if distant organ dysfunction is demonstrated (cardiovascular, neurologic, hematologic, respiratory, hepatic, renal). These staging systems can be used to better evaluate the indications for surgical treatment.

3.3 Treatment

Cholecystectomy has been the gold standard treatment for acute cholecystitis for many years, and traditionally it was accomplished several weeks after resolution of the acute phase (Figs. 3.3-3.7).

At the end of the 1970s the performance of cholecystectomy in the acute phase, during the same hospital admission, within 36-72 hours from the onset of symptoms (*early cholecystectomy*) gained the favor of many surgeons and in the following years several randomized controlled studies showed the benefits of this early approach, in terms of morbidity and mortality [30]. Reduced blood loss and operation time, lower complication rates and shorter hospital stay were also shown [31-33].

Early after the introduction of laparoscopic surgery, acute cholecystitis was considered a contraindication for laparoscopic cholecystectomy: the performance of a laparoscopic operation in the acute phase of a cholecystitis required experience and skills that were not common in the surgical community during those years, and a higher incidence of complication was found [34-36]. The difficulties related to the severe adhesion of the gallbladder to the surrounding tissues, thickness of the gallbladder wall limiting the handling of the organ, fibrosis of the gallbladder bed, identification and dissection of Calot's triangle structures in the presence of edema and adhesions could lead to several complications uncommon in the pre-laparoscopic era such as common bile duct, liver and bowel injuries.

Increased experience, gradual acquisition of the specific required skills, the awareness of the complications associated with laparoscopic cholecystectomy as well as the improvements in surgical instrumentation allowed us, in later years, to perform a laparoscopic cholecystectomy even in the most difficult

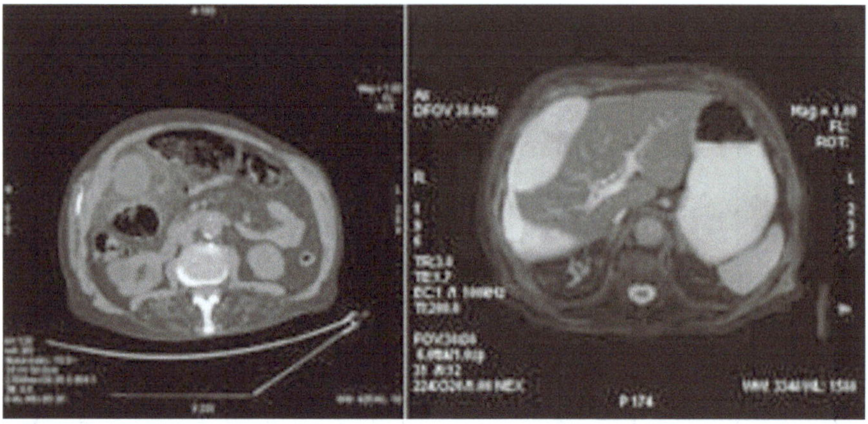

Fig. 3.3 A 62-year-old male patient. Pain in the right hypochondrium and fever (39.5°). Acute cholecystitis with filtration and bile collection (bilioma). Abdominal CT and MR: gallbladder perforation and collection under Glisson's capsule. Laparoscopic surgical treatment. Observation V. Mandalà

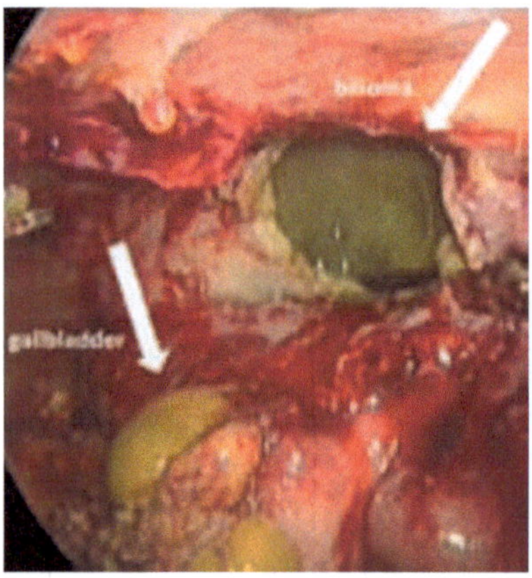

Fig. 3.4 Evacuation and opening of the bilioma

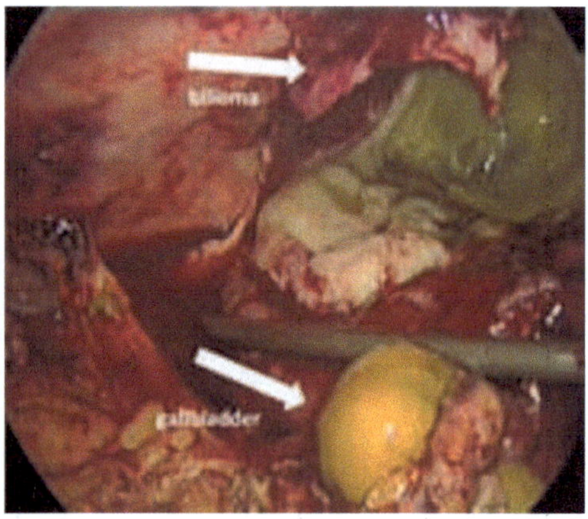

Fig. 3.5 Lavage and removal of the wall biloma

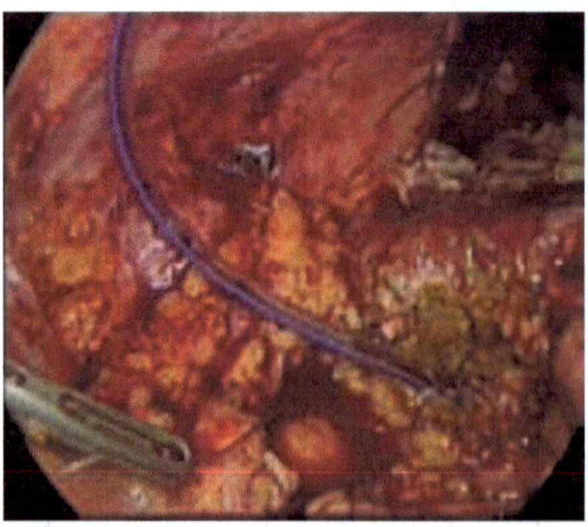

Fig. 3.6 Subtotal colecystectomy and transcystic drainage

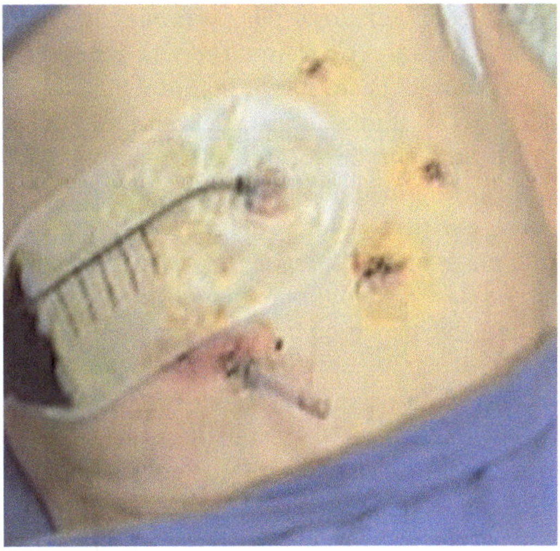

Fig. 3.7 Postoperative view

acute setting. Today laparoscopic cholecystectomy has proven to be safe and earlier reports of increased incidence of complication have not been confirmed. Two randomized trials [37, 38] and several comparative studies demonstrated faster recovery and shorter hospital stay after laparoscopic surgery for acute gallbladder disease. Recent population-based studies confirm that laparoscopic cholecystectomy is associated with lower morbidity, lower mortality, and shorter hospital stay [39, 40].

All available guidelines recommend laparoscopic cholecystectomy as the preferred approach for acute cholecystitis [19, 21, 23].

The best timing for laparoscopic cholecystectomy in acute cholecystitis is a relevant topic. During recent years several studies have compared early versus delayed laparoscopic cholecystectomy. In particular 5 meta-analyses [16, 30, 41-44,] examined the issue.

Even if the definition of the time interval for early or delayed surgery varies among the studies taken into consideration, all reviews reach the same conclusions: early laparoscopic cholecystectomy does not increase complication or conversion rates and reduces total hospital stay. The most feared complication in the earlier years – bile duct injury – was showed to be even higher in the delayed treated patients, but the difference was not statistically significant due to the limited statistical power of the trials.

The reviews also showed that 17.5% (range 13.9-25%) of patients included in the delayed surgery groups required urgent surgery during the interval period, for failure of conservative treatment or recurrent symptoms after discharge, and the overall conversion rate of this group was 45%.

One case series review addressed the issue of the amount of delay between onset of symptoms and surgery and examined its relation to the conversion rate, showing that the earlier the operation, the lower the risk of conversion.

The incidence of conversion is lowest (9.5%) if surgery is performed within 2 days from the onset of symptoms, and rises to 16.1% if surgery is done within 4 days. After that term the conversion rate is similar to that of delayed surgery (38.9%) [40]. However it needs to be pointed out that even though one recent observational study confirmed these findings [46], others did not [47-49] and one of the systematic reviews examined above [43] performed a subgroup analysis comparing data from the trials which included only patients treated less than four days from the onset of symptoms to those of the studies also including patients with a longer delay, and could not demonstrate a statistically significant difference between the two groups. Further studies could clarify this issue.

To what extent the findings discussed above and the related recommendations include also the severe forms of the disease (empyematous, gangrenous or perforated) is not clearly defined. The rate of severe cholecystitis is not specified in most studies and higher conversion rates have been reported when severe cholecystitis was treated by early laparoscopic surgery [50]; factors predicting the probability of conversion and complications have been analyzed, suggesting approaches based on a stricter selection of patients to subject to laparoscopic surgery or early conversion to open surgery [50, 51]. Alternative treatment modalities have also been proposed, such as subtotal cholecystectomy or cholecystostomy. The question whether laparoscopic treatment is related to a higher rate of complication in this particular setting or poses only a technical challenge with a higher conversion rate needs to be answered. One systematic review of available observational studies analyzed the surgical outcomes of laparoscopic cholecystectomy for severe acute cholecystitis and concluded that laparoscopic surgery is an acceptable indication even in the severe forms and no increase in local postoperative complications was shown. A threefold conversion rate has to be expected when approaching a severe cholecystitis [29]. However the review is limited by the absence of available controlled studies, and the need to include only those observational studies which clearly reported results of surgical treatment separately for severe acute cholecystitis and milder forms. It is likely that the conversion rate is at least partially related to the experience acquired by the surgical team and the probability of complications depends on a sound decision to convert to open surgery when the situation on the field is too difficult for the technical skills available. After all an adequate laparoscopic ability with extensive experience may overcome the limitation imposed by the angle of dissection and confined range of movements of the instruments, and by the reduced tactile feeling, and make the best use of the closer and more detailed operative laparoscopic view.

The overall increased complication rate, despite the absence of differences in local complications, observed in the examined studies about severe cholecystitis has been related to the systemic diseases associated with the severe form. This finding introduces the issue of laparoscopic cholecystectomy for acute cholecystitis in the presence of compromised general conditions and severe co-morbidity.

In fact patients with more co-morbid conditions and a high ASA classification are often excluded from receiving laparoscopic treatment fearing that the pathophysiologic changes due to laparoscopy and induction of CO_2 pneumoperitoneum could adversely affect the final outcome. On the other hand this particular subset of patients could receive larger benefits from the reduced surgical trauma, improved immunosuppression and postoperative respiratory function.

A particular group with a high incidence of co-morbid conditions is the aged population. The issue is relevant because the prevalence of gallstones significantly increases with age and cholelithiasis complications are also more common in this age group. The number of elderly patients with acute cholecystitis has been increasing over the years and earlier reports suggested a higher conversion rate for laparoscopic cholecystectomy in the elderly [52] and increased morbidity. Management of acute cholecystitis in the elderly is a real challenge due to significant co-morbidities, delayed presentation and increased morbidity associated with surgery. While delayed treatment can still be a viable option in these cases, omitted definitive surgery in the elderly has been associated with a 38% gallstone-related readmission rate in two years, as opposed to only 4% observed in patients who had cholecystectomy [53].

Alternative methods have been suggested for emergency treatment in high risk patients unfit for emergency surgery: conservative treatment [54], tube cholecystostomy followed by early laparoscopic surgery [55, 56], or by delayed surgery [18], and cholecystostomy not followed by surgery [57]. A systematic review of 53 observational studies about cholecystostomy in acute cholecystitis could find no evidence to support the recommendation of percutaneous drainage rather than straight early emergency cholecystectomy even in critically ill patients, and actually suggested that cholecystectomy seems to be a better alternative for treating acute cholecystitis in the elderly and/or critically ill population [58]. In their paper the authors examined a large number of studies, they warn about the low level of evidence of each of them and suggest that randomized controlled studies should be undertaken to clarify the issue. However, they found that therapeutic failure, recurring cholecystitis or procedural complications of percutaneous cholecystostomy led to emergency surgery in 4.5% of patients and overall mortality rates were much worse for patients treated with percutaneous cholecystostomy when compared to the outcomes for acute cholecystectomy published in series with similar populations.

While the above described review does not make a specific distinction between laparoscopic and open cholecystectomy in the elderly or critically ill, some comparative studies examined laparoscopic versus open surgery for acute cholecystitis in these patients and showed a reduction in the hospital stay [59-61] and morbidity either unchanged [59] or improved [60, 61] in the laparoscopic treatment groups.

3.4 Surgical Technique

A traditional retrograde infundibular laparoscopic approach has been used for the dissection of Calot's triangle and separation of the gallbladder from the liver bed in acute cholecystitis. However, the critical-view-of-safety technique described by Strasberg has been increasingly used and has replaced the infundibular approach in many surgical practices [64, 65] in particular in the acute setting.

If the identification and dissection of the Calot's triangle structures has been made difficult by adhesions or inflammation, a laparoscopic *fundus first* anterograde approach used by many surgeons to avoid common bile duct injury [65, 66].

Selective use of intraoperative cholangiography is commonly adopted to clarify the anatomy or a suspicion of common bile duct stone. Modifications of the procedure are included when necessary (decompression of the gallbladder, introduction of an additional cannula, sutures to control the cystic duct).

Variations of the technique have been proposed including three-port technique [67], and single port [68], however no controlled trials comparing these techniques to standard laparoscopy for acute cholecystitis have been published. A randomized trial of mini-laparoscopy versus conventional laparoscopy showed no significant difference between the two techniques [69].

In cases where the local conditions are particularly hostile due to intense inflammation and increased risk of damage to Calot triangle structures, subtotal cholecystectomy has been advocated as an alternative solution [70] and it has been included in the surgical strategies to reduce conversion rates without increasing complications [71].

Many surgeons find the use of ultrasonic dissection particularly useful to face the challenge of laparoscopic cholecystectomy for acute cholecystitis: the ability of this particular technology to divide tenacious adhesions, intense fibrosis and to achieve hemostasis in the areas of neovascularization, allow for safer dissection in the acute setting. A randomized clinical trial of traditional electrocautery versus ultrasonic dissection demonstrated that operative time in laparoscopic cholecystectomy performed for acute cholecystitis is significantly shorter if ultrasonic technology is used [72]. A prospective observational study confirmed this finding and showed a reduction in conversion rates for acute cholecystitis operated laparoscopically with ultrasonic dissection [73]. An Italian randomized trial is being conducted on this topic to clarify these observations [74].

3.5 Authors' Surgical Series

We analyze the experience of two Italian surgical centers with different types of patient recruitment: a ten year data report from a large urban area hospital (Palermo) and a series from a smaller suburban hospital (Civita Castellana – Viterbo).

In Villa Sofia Hospital (Palermo, Dept of General and Emergency Surgery) 1487 patients underwent cholecystectomy from January 2000 to December 2010, in 412 cases surgery was done for acute cholecystitis. The age of the patients ranged from 20 to 86 years, the mean age was 62.9 (>80 years old: 35 patients, 8.5%), and the sex distribution was 233 females (56.7%) and 179 males (43.3%).

Laparoscopic cholecystectomy (VLC) was performed in 354 patients (84.9%) as follows: VLC: 304 (85.8%), robotic assisted laparoscopy: 11(3.1%), subtotal VLC: 39 (11.1%).

Open procedures were performed in 45 patients (11.3%) with 6 sub total open cholecystectomies; 9 VLC procedures were converted to open cholecystectomy. A subhepatic drain was left in all patients.

Nine patients underwent US-guided percutaneous cholecystostomy (2.3%) and 4 video-assisted cholecystostomy (1.2%). The following complications occurred in the open procedure: 6 cases of sub phrenic abscess (13.3%), 12 cases of surgical wound infections (26.6%) and 3 cases of pneumonia (6.6%). In the sub total laparoscopic cholecystectomy series there were 3 cases of subphrenic abscesses (7.7%), 1 case of pneumonia (2.6%), 1 bile leak (2.6%) and 6 surgical wound complications (15.3%). There was one death from myocardial infarction (0.28%) after VLC.

From January 2010 to April 2011, 111 patients underwent laparoscopic cholecystectomy at the Andosilla Hospital (Civita Castellana, VT - Italy). A total of 56 VLC were performed for acute cholecystitis. There were 6 patients >80 years of age (10%). No procedure was started as open cholecystectomy and only in one case was a conversion from laparoscopic to open surgery necessary (1.7%). No percutaneous cholecystostomy was done. One elderly patient (83 years old) with multiple cardiac and respiratory co-morbidities died from myocardial infarction (mortality rate 1.7%) on the fourth postoperative day.

In the series from Villa Sofia in Palermo, open procedures were prevalent in the first three years while laparoscopic procedures were increasingly represented in the last five years. Open procedures showed a higher complication rate. The conversion rate decreased with increasing surgical expertise and in the last year there were no cases of conversion. The nine laparoscopic cholecystectomies converted to an open procedure were performed during the first six years of this data collection.

The hospital in Civita Castellana is a community-based suburban hospital serving a district with a population of about 55,000. The surgical team is small but well trained. About one half of the cholecystectomies were performed for acute cholecystitis. All cholecystectomies were laparoscopic. This unselected consecutive series shows a very low conversion rate. A small, well motivated, expert laparoscopic team can achieve excellent results in a small community hospital.

3.6 Conclusions

Laparoscopic surgery for acute cholecystitis may be challenging due to technical reasons as well as higher incidence of co-morbid disease in the affected population. The more severe forms of the disease imply difficult technical issues and specific risks related to sepsis and distant organ dysfunction. Longer life expectancy along with a prevalence of cholelithiasis sharply increasing with age does not allow us to ignore the request for minimally invasive treatment in the elderly and the concern for appropriate therapeutic strategies in this age group will grow in the future. The increasing awareness of possible complications of laparoscopic surgery along with the acquisition of skills and experience in the surgical community have made laparoscopic cholecystectomy to be considered the gold standard for acute cholecystitis even in critical situations and the literature supporting the evidence of laparoscopic indications is becoming increasingly available.

References

1. Brewer BJ, Golden GT, Hitch DC at al (1976) Abdominal pain. An analysis of 1000 consecutive cases in a University Hospital emergency room. Am J Surg 131:219-223
2. Reiss R, Deutsch AA (1993) State of the art in the diagnosis and management of acute cholecystitis. Dig Dis 11:55-64
3. Yasutoshi K, Tadahiro T, Yoshifumi K et al (2007) Definitions, pathophysiology, and epidemiology of acute cholangitis and cholecystitis: Tokyo Guidelines J Hepatobiliary Pancreat Surg 14(1):15-26
4. Williamson RC (1988) Acalculous disease of the gall bladder. Gut 29:860-72
5. Barie PS, Fischer E (1995) Acute acalculous cholecystitis. J Am Coll Surg 180:232-44
6. Cello JP (1998) AIDS-Related biliary tract disease. Gastrointest Endosc Clin North Am 8(4):963
7. Janzon L, Aspelin P, Eriksson S et al (1985) Ultrasonographic screening for gallstone disease in middle-aged women. Detection rate, symptoms, and biochemical features. Scand J Gatroenterol 20:706-710
8. Jørgensen T (1987) Prevalence of gallstones in a Danish population. Am J Epidemiol 126:912-921
9. Muhrbeck O, Ahlberg J (1995) Prevalence of gallstones in a Swedish population. Scand J Gastroenterol 30:1125-1128
10. Attili AF, Carulli N, Roda E et al (1995) Epidemiology of gallstone disease in Italy; prevalence data of the multicenter Italian study on cholelithiasis (MICOL). Am J Epidemiol 141:158-65
11. Shaffer EA (2006) Epidemiology of gallbladder stone disease. Best Practices and Research Clinical Gastroenterology. 20(6):981-996
12. Halldestam I, Enell EL, Kullman E, Borch K (2004) Development of symptoms and complications in individuals with asymptomatic gallstones. Br J Surg 91:734-738
13. National Institutes of Health, U.S. Department of Health and Human Services. Opportunities and Challenges in Digestive Diseases Research: Recommendations of the National Commission on Digestive Diseases. Bethesda, MD: National Institutes of Health; 2009. NIH Publication 08–6514. http://catalog.niddk.nih.gov/detail.cfm?id=1252 Accessed 9 may 2011
14. Ministero della Salute (2010) Ricoveri, diagnosi, interventi effettuati e durata delle degenze di tutti gli ospedali. http://www.salute.gov.it/ricoveriOspedalieri/ric_informazioni/default.jsp. Accessed 9 May 2011

15. David GG, Al-Sarira AA, Wilmott S et al (2008) Management of acute gallbladder disease in England. Br J Surg 95:472-476
16. Gurusamy K, Samraj K, Gluud C, Wilson E, Davidson BR (2010) Meta-analysis of randomized controlled trials on the safety and effectiveness of early versus delayed laparoscopic cholecystectomy for acute cholecystitis. Br J Surg 97(2):141-150
17. Ainsworth AP, Adamsen S, Rosenberg J.(2007) Surgery for acute cholecystitis in Denmark. Scand J Gastroenterol 42:648-51
18. Borzellino G., de Manzoni G, Ricci F, Gastaldini G, Guglielmi A., Cordiano C (1999) Emergency cholecystostomy and subsequent cholecystectomy for acute gallstones cholecystitis in the elderly. Br J Surg 86:1521-1525
19. Sauerland S, Agresta F, Bergamaschi R et al (2006) Laparoscopy for abdominal emergencies: evidence based guidelines of the European Association for Endoscopic Surgery. Surg Endosc 20(1):14-29
20. Hirota M, Takada T, Kawarada Y et al (2007) Diagnostic criteria and severity assessment of acute cholecystitis: Tokyo Guidelines. J Hepatobiliary Pancreat Surg. 14(1):78-82
21. Yamashita Y, Takada T, Kawarada Y et al (2007) Surgical treatment of patients with acute cholecystitis: Tokyo Guidelines. J Hepatobiliary Pancreat Surg. 14(1):91-97
22. Yasuda H, Takada T, Kawarada Y et al (2007) Unusual cases of acute cholecystitis and cholangitis: Tokyo Guidelines.J Hepatobiliary Pancreat Surg. 14(1):98-113
23. Overby DW, Apelgren KN, Richardson W, Fanelli R (2010) SAGES guidelines for the clinical application of laparoscopic biliary tract surgery. Surg Endosc 24(10):2368-2386
24. Trowbridge RL, Rutkowski NK, Shojania KG (2003) Does this patient have acute cholecystitis? J Am Med Assoc 289:80-86
25. Juvonen T, Kiviniemi H, Niemela O, Kairaluoma MI (1992) Diagnostic accuracy of ultrasonography and C-reactive protein concentra-tion in acute cholecystitis: a prospective clinical study. Eur J Surg 1992;158:365-369
26. Hanbidge AE, Buckler PM, O'Malley ME, Wilson SR (2004) From the RSNA refresher courses: imaging evaluation for acute pain in the right upper quadrant. Radiographics 24:1117-1135
27. Smith EA, Dillman JR, Elsayes KM, Menias CO, Bude RO (2009) Cross-sectional imaging of acute and chronic gallbladder inflammatory disease. AJR Am J Roentgenol 192:188-196
28. Park MS, Yu JS, Kim YH, Kim MJ et al (1998) Acute cholecystitis: comparison of MR cholangiography and US Radiology. 209:781-785
29. Borzellino G, Sauerland S, Minicozzi AM et al (2008) Laparoscopic cholecystectomy for severe acute cholecystitis. A meta-analysis of results. Surg Endosc 22(1):8-15
30. Papi C, Catarci M, D'Ambrosjo L et al (2004) Timing of cholecystectomy for acute calculous cholecystitis: a meta-analysis. Am J Gastroenterol 99:147-155
31. Lahtinen J, Alhava EM, Aukee S (1978) Acute cholecystitits treated by early and delayed surgery. A controlled clinical trial. Scand J Gastroenterol 13:673-678
32. Jarvinen HJ, Hastbacka J (1980) Early cholecystectomy for acute cholecystitis: a prospective randomized study. Ann Surg 191:501-505
33. Norrby S, Herlin P, Holmin T, Sjodahl R, Tagesson C (1983) Early or delayed cholecystectomy in acute cholecystitis? A clinical trial. Br J Surg 70:163-165
34. Cushieri A, Dubois F, Mouiel J et al (1991) The European experience with laparoscopic cholecystectomy. Am J Surg 161:385-387
35. Kum CK, Eypasch E, Lefering R et al (1996) Laparoscopic cholecystectomy for acute cholecystitis: is it really safe? World J Surg 20:43-49
36. Russell JC, Walsh SJ, Mattie AS, Lynch JT (1996) Bile duct injuries, 1989-1993. A statewide experience. Arch Surg 131:382-388
37. Kiviluoto T, Siren J, Luukkonen P, Kivilaakso E (1998) Randomised trial of laparoscopic versus open cholecystectomy for acute and gangrenous cholecystitis. Lancet 351:321-325
38. Johansson M, Thune A, Nelvin L et al (2005) Randomized clinical trial of open versus laparoscopic cholecystectomy in the treatment of acute cholecystitis. Br J Surg 92:44-49
39. Csikesz N, Ricciardi R, Tseng JF, Shah SA (2008) Current status of surgical management of acute cholecystitis in the United States. World J Surg 32(10):2230-2236

40. Zacks SL, Sandler RS, Rutledge R, Brown RS (2002) A population-based cohort study comparing laparoscopic cholecystectomy and open cholecystectomy. Am J Gastroenterol 97:334-340
41. Shikata S, Noguchi Y, Fukui T (2005) Early ersus delayed cholecystectomy for acute cholecystitis: a meta-analysis of randomized controlled trials. Surg Today 35:553-560
42. Lau H, Lo Y, Patil NG, Yuen WK (2006) Early versus delayed-interval laparoscopic cholecystectomy for acute cholecystitis. A metaanalysis. Surg Endosc 20:82-87
43. Gurusamy KS, Samraj K (2006) Early versus delayed laparoscopic cholecystectomy for acute cholecystitis. Chochrane Database Syst Rev (4):CD005440
44. Siddiqui T, MacDonald A, Chong PS, Jenkins JT (2008) Early versus delayed laparoscopic cholecystectomy for acute cholecystitis: a meta-analysis of randomized clinical trials. Am J Surg 195(1):40-47
45. Hadad SM, Vaidya JS, Baker L et al (2007) Delay from symptom onset increases the conversion rate in laparoscopic cholecystectomy for acute cholecystitis World J Surg 31:1298-1301
46. Catani M, De Milito R, Romagnoli F et al (2008) The best timing of surgery in laparoscopic cholecystectomy for acute cholecystitis: when and how is to be performed. Hepatogastroenterology 55(88):1993-1996
47. Low JK, Barrow P, Owera A, Ammori BJ (2007) Timing of laparoscopic cholecystectomy for acute cholecystitis: evidence to support a proposal for an early interval surgery. Am Surg 73(11):1188-1192
48. Popkharitov A (2008) Laparoscopic cholecystectomy for acute cholecystitis. Langenbecks Arch Surg 393(6):935-941
49. Farooq T, Buchanan G, Manda V, Kennedy R, Ockrim J (2009) Is early laparoscopic cholecystectomy safe after the "safe period"? J Laparoendosc Adv Surg Tech A 19(4):471-474
50. Cox MR, Wilson TG, Luck AJ, Jeans PL, Padbury RT, Toouli J (1993) Laparoscopic cholecystectomy for acute inflammation of the gallbladder. Ann Surg 21:630-634
51. Eldar S, Sabo E, Nash E, Abrahamson J, Matter I (1998) Laparoscopic cholecystectomy for the various types of gallbladder inflammation: a prospective trial. Surg Laparosc Endosc 8(3):200-207
52. Fried GM, Barkun JS, Sigman HH et al (1994) Factors determining conversion to laparotomy in patients undergoing laparoscopic cholecystectomy. Am J Surg 167:35-41
53. Riall TS, Zhang D, Townsend CM Jr, Kuo YF, Goodwin JS (2010) Failure to perform cholecystectomy for acute cholecystitis in elderly patients is associated with increased morbidity, mortality, and cost. J Am Coll Surg 210(5):668-77, 677-9
54. Vetrhus M, Soreide O, Nesvik I, Sondenaa K (2003) Acute cholecystitis: delayed surgery or observation. A randomized clinical trial. Scand J Gastroenterol 38:985-990
55. Akyürek N, Salman B, Yüksel O et al (2005) Management of acute calculous cholecystitis in high-risk patients: percutaneous cholecystotomy followed by early laparoscopic cholecystectomy. Surg Laparosc Endosc Percutan Tech. 15(6):315-320
56. Macrì A, Scuderi G, Saladino E et al (2006) Acute gallstone cholecystitis in the elderly: treatment with emergency ultrasonographic percutaneous cholecystostomy and interval laparoscopic cholecystectomy. Surg Endosc 20(1):88-91
57. Kim HJ, Lee SK, Kim MH et al (2000) Safety and usefulness of percutaneous transhepatic cholecystoscopy examination in high-risk surgical patients with acute cholecystitis. Gastrointest Endosc 52(5):645-649
58. Pessaux P, Regenet N, Tuech JJ et al (2001) Laparoscopic versus open cholecystectomy: A prospective comparative study in the elderly with acute cholecystitis. Surg Laparosc Endosc Percutan Tech 11:252-255
59. Winbladh A, Gullstrand P, Svanvik J, Sandström P (2009) Systematic review of cholecystostomy as a treatment option in acute cholecystitis. HPB 11(3):183-193
60. Lujan JA,Sanchez-Bueno F,Parrilla P et al (1998) Laparoscopic vs. open cholecystectomy in patients aged 65 and older. Surg Laparosc Endosc Percutan Tech 8(3):208-210
61. Chau CH, Tang CN, Siu WT, Ha JP, Li MK (2002) Laparoscopic cholecystectomy versus open

cholecystectomy in elderly patients with acute cholecystitis: retrospective study. Hong Kong Med J 8:394-399
62. Massie MT, Massie LB, Marrangoni AG, D'Amico FJ, Sell HW (1993) Advantages of laparoscopic cholecystectomy in the elderly and in patients with high ASA classifications. J Laparoendosc Surg 3:467-476
63. Buddingh KT, Hofker HS, Ten Cate Hoedemaker HO, van Dam GM, Ploeg RJ, Nieuwenhuijs VB (2011) Safety measures during cholecystectomy: results of a nationwide survey. World J Surg 35(6):1235-1241
64. Casillas RA, Yegiyants S, Collins JC (2008) Early laparoscopic cholecystectomy is the preferred management of acute cholecystitis. Arch Surg 143(6):533-537
65. Wang YC, Yang HR, Chung PK, Jeng LB, Chen RJ (2006) Role of fundus-first laparoscopic cholecystectomy in the management of acute cholecystitis in elderly patients. J Laparoendosc Adv Surg Tech A 16(2):124-127
66. Kelly MD (2009) Laparoscopic retrograde (fundus first) cholecystectomy. BMC Surg 11:19 Doi:10.1186/1471-2482-9-19
67. Al-Azawi D, Houssein N, Rayis AB, McMahon D, Hehir DJ (2007) Three-port versus four-port laparoscopic cholecystectomy in acute and chronic cholecystitis. BMC Surg 13:8. Doi: 10.1186/1471-2482-7-8
68. Elsey JK, Feliciano DV (2010) Initial experience with single-incision laparoscopic cholecystectomy. J Am Coll Surg 210(5):620-624, 624-626
69. Hsieh CH (2003) Early laparoscopic cholecystectomy in patients with acute cholecystitis. Am J Surg 185:344-348
70. Soleimani M, Mehrabi A, Mood ZA et al (2007) Partial cholecystectomy as a safe and viable option in the emergency treatment of complex acute cholecystitis: a case series and review of the literature. Am Surg 73(5):498-507
71. Low SW, Iyer SG, Chang SK, Mak KS, Lee VT, Madhavan K (2009) Laparoscopic cholecystectomy for acute cholecystitis: safe implementation of successful strategies to reduce conversion rates. Surg Endosc 23(11):2424-2429
72. Cengiz Y, Jänes A, Grehn A, Israelsson LA (2005) Randomized trial of traditional dissection with electrocautery versus ultrasonic fundus-first dissection in patients undergoing laparoscopic cholecystectomy. Br J Surg 92(7):810-813
73. Catena F, Ansaloni L, Di Saverio S, Gazzotti F, Coccolini F, Pinna AD (2009) Prospective analysis of 101 consecutive cases of laparoscopic cholecystectomy for acute cholecystitis operated with harmonic scalpel. Surg Laparosc Endosc Percutan Tech 19(4):312-316
74. Catena F, Ansaloni L, Di Saverio S, Gazzotti F, Coccolini F, Pinna AD (2009) The HAC Trial (Harmonic for Acute Cholecystitis) Study. Randomized, double-blind, controlled trial of Harmonic(H) versus Monopolar Diathermy (M) for laparoscopic cholecystectomy (LC) for acute cholecystitis (AC) in adults. Trials 26;10:34

Suggested Readings

Sauerland S, Agresta F, Bergamaschi R, Borzellino G, Budzynski A, Champault G, Fingerhut A, Isla A, Johansson M, Lundorff P (2006) Laparoscopy for abdominal emergencies. Evidence-based guidelines of the European Association for Endoscopic Surgery. Surg Endosc 20:14–29

Agresta F, Ansaloni L, Baiocchi L, Bergamini C, Campanile FB, Carlucci M, Cocorullo G, Corradi A, Franzato B, Lupo M, Mandalà V, Mirabella A, Pernazza G, Piccoli M, Staudacher C, Vettoretto N, Zago M, Lettieri E, Levati A, Pietrini D, Scaglione M, De Masi S, De Placido G, Francucci M, Rasi M, Scaramuzza G, Del Favero AL (2011) Consensus Development Conference of the Società Italiana Chirurgia Endoscopica e nuove tecnologie (SICE); Associazione Chirurghi Ospedalieri Italiani (ACOI); Società Italiana di Chirurgia (SIC); Società Italiana Chirurgia d'Urgenza e Trauma (SICUT), Società Italiana Chirurghi dell'Ospedalità Privata (SICOP) and the European Association for Endoscopic Surgery (EAES). In press

Acute Pancreatitis

4

Carlo Staudacher, Gianpaolo Balzano, Nicolò Pecorelli
and Vincenzo Mandalà

4.1 Introduction

4.1.1 Epidemiology

The incidence of acute pancreatitis (AP) has increased over the last two decades to become a growing problem both in the United States and Europe [1, 2]. Between 1994 and 2001, the incidence of first-time attack in California increased from 33 to 44 per 100,000 adults [2] and at present AP accounts for more than 200,000 hospital admissions every year in the USA [3]. Data from the Italian Ministry of Health register show a total of 20,174 admissions for AP in Italy in 2005.

Apart from the increasing overall incidence, the rate of severe acute pancreatitis (SAP) has remained stable. In 80% of patients, AP is mild and resolves without serious morbidity, with a brief hospitalization, but up to 20% of patients develop a severe form, complicated by substantial morbidity and mortality [4]. This distribution was confirmed in a recent multicentre survey involving 1,173 patients from 56 Italian hospitals equally distributed throughout the country. Considering the Atlanta classification system [5], 1,006 patients (85.8%) were defined as having mild AP and 167 (14.2%) as experiencing the severe form. In the same survey mortality for AP occurred in 3.1% of the patients, mostly from multiple organ failure due to infected pancreatic necrosis [6].

C. Staudacher (✉)
Head of Department of Surgical Sciences
San Raffaele Scientific Institute
Milan, Italy

V. Mandalà, *The Role of Laparoscopy in Emergency Abdominal Surgery*,

Table 4.1 Ranson's criteria for severity of acute pancreatitits

At admission	During initial 48 h
Age > 55 yrs	Hematocrit decrease of more than 0.10
White blood cell count < 16×10^9/L	Blood urea nitrogen increases by > 5 mg/dL
Lactate dehydrogenase > 350 U/L	Calcium < 8 mg/dL
Aspartate aminotransferase > 250 U/L	PaO_2 < 60 mmHg
Glucose > 200 mg/dL	Base deficit > 4 mEq/L
	Fluid sequestration > 6 L

Predicted severe acute pancreatitis indicated by a total score ≥3, with 1 point for each positive factor.

4.1.2 Assessment of Severity

A crucial aspect in the management of this disease is a prompt assessment of severity. Although most patients have a mild episode of AP, it is difficult to identify patients who are at risk of developing severe disease on admission to the hospital. Severity of AP is defined by the presence or absence of organ failure, local complications, or both. Recognized markers of the risk of SAP include specific laboratory values that measure systemic inflammatory response (e.g. C-reactive protein) and multi-factorial scoring systems based on clinical and laboratory findings which assess inflammation or organ failure (such as Ranson's score, Glasgow Score and the Acute Physiology and Chronic Health Evaluation score - APACHE II). Furthermore, contrast-enhanced CT scan imaging performed at least 48 hours after the onset of AP is useful for evaluating disease severity, as it gives an indication of the degree of necrotic tissue [7]. Once a predicted SAP has been identified, the patient should be referred to a specialized centre for pancreatic diseases [8]: in these cases patients could require intensive care support, while decision-making about invasive treatment (adequate timing and choice of treatment) requires special expertise (Tables 4.1, 4.2).

4.2 The Role of Surgery in Acute Pancreatitis

There are three potential indications for surgery in acute pancreatitis, here listed in order of frequency: (1) the presence of gallstones; (2) pancreatic necrosis (mainly infected necrosis); and (3) abdominal compartment syndrome (ACS). Minimally invasive surgery plays different roles, according to the different indications and the severity of the acute attack: most cholecystectomies can be performed laparoscopically, and even in the setting of necrosectomy, minimally invasive surgery is gaining increasing surgical attention. On the other hand, laparoscopy is formally contraindicated in cases of ACS.

Table 4.2 Balthazar's CT severity index

CT grade	CT finding	Points
A	Normal pancreas	0
B	Pancreatic enlargement	1
C	Pancreatic inflammation and/or peripancreatic fat	2
D	Single peripancreatic fluid collection	3
E	Two or more fluid collections and/or retroperitoneal air	4
Necrosis	**Points**	
None	0	
< 30 %	2	
30–50 %	4	
> 50%	6	
CT severity index (CT grade + necrosis score)	**Complications**	**Mortality**
0–3	8%	3%
4–6	35%	6%
7–10	92%	17%

4.2.1 Gallstone-Associated Acute Pancreatitis

Biliary tract disease is the most common etiology for AP in the Western world. In the recent multicentre study performed by the Italian Association for the Study of the Pancreas (AISP) biliary forms accounted for 69.3% of cases [6].

In gallstone-associated AP, the pancreatitis is usually mild and self-limited. The treatment should initially be supportive with subsequent laparoscopic cholecystectomy to prevent recurrent attacks. Although available guidelines do not address the issue whether cholecystectomy should be performed by open or laparoscopic approach, they all suggest that surgery should be performed as soon as the patient has recovered and during the same hospital admission [9, 10]. A recent randomized controlled trial (RCT) found that laparoscopic cholecystectomy performed within 48 hours of admission, regardless of the resolution of abdominal pain or laboratory abnormalities, resulted in a shorter hospital length of stay with no apparent impact on the technical difficulty of the procedure or perioperative complication rate [11]. Furthermore there is evidence to suggest that delaying cholecystectomy increases technical difficulties during dissection [12]. Nonetheless the actual timing of surgery often contradicts the suggestions of the guidelines. In clinical practice there is a tendency to delay cholecystectomy until after complete resolution of pain and normalization of laboratory values; patients are frequently discharged after the acute attack and readmitted at a later time to undergo elective cholecystectomy, increasing the risk of gallstone-related events including recurrent AP [13]. A recent prospective multicenter study on the surgical treatment of acute pancreatitis in Italy confirmed poor compliance of clinical practice with published guidelines: of 593 patients with mild pancreatitis of biliary origin and indication to cholecystectomy, only 36% underwent the operation during the same admission [14].

In addition, clearance of potential common bile duct (CBD) stones is crucial to prevent further recurrent attacks. Ideally, when CBD stones are suspected, this should be confirmed preoperatively by either endoscopic ultrasonography (EUS) or magnetic resonance cholangiography (MRC). Both techniques carry high sensitivity and specificity (over 90%) preventing the risk of complications due to unnecessary CBD exploration by either endoscopic retrograde cholangiopancreatography (ERCP) or intraoperatively [15, 16]. If diagnosis of CBD stones is confirmed, it can be managed both by preoperative ERCP [17], and laparoscopic CBD clearance during cholecystectomy [18]. Two meta-analyses showed no differences when preoperative ERCP was compared to intraoperative removal of CBD stones [19, 20]. The choice of treatment should be determined by local availability and expertise, since laparoscopic CBD exploration requires significant surgical skill.

In cases of severe acute biliary pancreatitis, patients are at a high risk of organ failure and death, especially in the early phase of the disease. There is consensus that cholecystectomy in severe forms should be delayed until the pancreatitis has resolved with normalization of the inflammatory response and clinical recovery, since early operation is associated with a higher complication rate [8, 10, 21, 22].

Though it is not among the aims of this chapter, here is a short note on the indication to early ERCP in severe forms: while it is clear that cholangitis should always be treated by endoscopic drainage of the bile duct, the role of ERCP for the treatment of cholestasis in SAP is still controversial [23]. In accordance with the American College of Gastroenterology guidelines [24], we suggest that ERCP and biliary sphincterotomy be performed (preferably within 24 h of admission) for patients with predicted severe biliary pancreatitis in the presence of cholangitis and/or retained common bile duct stones. In a recent RCT by the Dutch Acute Pancreatitis Group, early ERCP was associated with a significantly reduced risk of clinically relevant complications in patients with predicted SAP with concurrent cholestasis, whereas in patients without cholestasis, there were no beneficial effects [25].

4.2.2 Necrotic Pancreatitis

Recently published data report that the severe form accounts for about 15% of 272,000 patients hospitalized each year due to acute pancreatitis in the United States [3]. SAP, as defined by the Atlanta Symposium criteria [5], is characterized by organ dysfunction, which is usually associated with the development of pancreatic necrosis which reaches its maximum extent within the first 4 days after the onset of symptoms.

The presence of necrosis is associated with a high mortality rate, around 17%. Initially, the necrosis is sterile, and if it remains so, mortality is approximately 12%, but when necrosis infection occurs, it carries a high risk of sepsis and multiple organ failure, raising the mortality rate to 30% [24]. Infection of necrotic tissue usually takes place 2 to 3 weeks after the onset of symptoms [26, 27], and occurs in 40 to 70% of cases [21]. When infection of necrotic tissue is suspected due to deterioration of clinical conditions, increase of inflammation markers or persistent organ failure, CT-guided percutaneous aspiration of necrotic tissue with Gram's stain and culture is recommended [8, 21, 25]. Alternatively, even direct CT evidence of gas in the retroperitoneum may be diagnostic of infected pancreatic necrosis [21, 24, 28].

Since Bradley first introduced the concept of conservative treatment in non-infected pancreatic necrosis in 1991, showing that the mortality rate for nonoperative management of patients with sterile necrotizing pancreatitis was inferior to surgical mortality rates [29], the indications for surgical intervention in sterile pancreatic necrosis has dropped consistently. Currently, as recommended by all available guidelines, patients with sterile pancreatic necrosis should be managed conservatively and undergo intervention only in selected cases, such as those patients with multiorgan failure who do not improve despite maximal therapy in the intensive care unit [8].

In patients with infected necrosis there is agreement that surgical intervention directed toward mechanical removal of as much necrotic tissue as possible, with debridement of all cavities containing necrotic material, is mandatory. However, the timing of intervention is crucial, since an early operation does not allow a complete demarcation of the tissues to be removed. Postponing surgical intervention allows the immune system to encapsulate the necrotic tissue, thus technically facilitating necrosectomy and potentially reducing mortality. This strategy is supported by evidence from a RCT comparing intervention within 72 h of onset with operation after 12 days, showing a reduction in mortality from 56% to 27% in patients who underwent late operation [30]. A later retrospective study demonstrated that necrosectomy for documented or suspected infected acute necrotizing pancreatitis performed after 29 days is associated with even lower mortality when compared with interventions in the first 2 weeks and from weeks 2 to 4 [31]. However, in these patients an increase in fungal colonization and resistant microorganisms is to be expected, owing to the increased use of antibiotics. Consequently, current guidelines recommend delaying surgery in patients with infected pancreatic necrosis at least until the third week after admission [8, 21].

Despite consensus on optimal timing for surgical intervention in SAP, adherence to these guidelines in clinical practice is poor. In the above cited Italian multicentre trial, 29 out of 167 patients (17.4%) with SAP were operated. Surprisingly, surgery was performed at a median of 2 days (range 0–64 days) after the onset of pancreatitis. MOF and infected necrosis were reported to be the main indications for surgery; mortality was higher in patients with early surgery (during the first 5 days after onset of symptoms), confirming the need for delaying intervention [14].

When invasive treatment of necrosis is indicated, the open approach has been considered the gold standard until very recent times. Over the years different techniques have been employed including necrosectomy with closed continuous irrigation of the lesser sac and retroperitoneum via indwelling catheters [26, 32], necrosectomy with open packing and planned re-laparotomy [33] or necrosectomy with closed drainage without irrigation [32, 34]. Although there has been a reduction in mortality rates especially with the development of open packing with repeated re-laparotomies and the use of prolonged postoperative lavage techniques, even in specialist units the mortality rate for infected necrosis is reported to be as high as 39% [24, 35–38]. Moreover, this invasive approach carries high rates of complications, up to 95%, and a risk of long-term pancreatic insufficiency [32, 36].

In this scenario, since the late 1990s, due to rapid advances in technology and the application of laparoscopy in an increasing number of surgical procedures, minimally invasive approaches to necrotic tissue with different drainage and necrosectomy techniques have been developed. These techniques were initially adopted in patients with infected pancreatic necrosis unfit to undergo prompt open surgical debridement [38], but in recent years their use has began to be extended to all patients because of the persistently high mortality and morbidity rate of the traditional open approach. These approaches find their rationale in the evidence that minimally invasive surgery provokes less surgical trauma and reduced activation of the inflammatory response than equivalent open surgery, and experimental studies suggest that local sepsis and the inflammatory response may be lessened by a minimally invasive rather than an open technique [31, 39].

In 1998 Freeney et al. [40] first reported a series of patients with infected necrotizing pancreatitis treated by CT-guided percutaneous drainage with encouraging results: in 47% of the patients drainage was successful, with no need of further intervention, while in another 27% of the patients the drain allowed sepsis to be controlled and surgery to be delayed, thus avoiding an emergency procedure in a group of critically ill patients. Mortality was low with an overall rate of 12%. Since then, several studies have reported the use of percutaneous drainage alone or in association with the use of accessories such as snares and baskets for debridement [41]. Although most studies reported a high success rate with low mortality, a common drawback was the high rate of fistula formation and the need for frequent catheter care and repeated procedures. In addition, single institution expertise intuitively plays a major role in determining the feasibility of the drainage.

Another approach described in recent years is the endoscopic (transgastric or transduodenal) access for drainage/debridement of necrosis in carefully selected patients [42, 43]. Recently the introduction of EUS guidance and Doppler imaging in order to avoid blood vessels has provided a safer approach. Endoscopic treatment may avoid the formation of external fistulae, but the need for necrosis to be organized (walled-off) and the inability to evacuate large areas of non-liquefied necrotic debris represent limitations for this technique [44].

Laparoscopic debridement and necrosectomy was first proposed in 1996 by Gagner [45], who used three alternative laparoscopic approaches: transgastric, retrogastric-retrocolic debridement, and a full retroperitoneoscopic technique. Other reports using similar techniques followed [46–49]. The largest series of transperitoneal laparoscopic debridement is reported by Parekh [47], who adopted a hand-assisted laparoscopic technique for pancreatic necrosis debridement in nineteen patients. He described an infracolic approach to access the lesser sac through the transverse mesocolon with an 81% success rate, low mortality (11%) and no major wound complications or external bowel fistulae.

The traditional transperitoneal laparoscopic approach compared to other minimally invasive techniques has the advantage of allowing access to areas inaccessible by a percutaneous drainage or an endoscope, including the right and the left paracolic gutters, the perinephric space, the retroduodenal space, and the root of the mesentery, permitting complete removal of the sequestrum. On the other hand we can argue that induction of pneumoperitoneum may have adverse effects in critically ill patients with hemodynamic instability. Furthermore the procedure carries a higher risk of infection transmission through the peritoneal cavity and bowel injury during surgery.

To avoid such risks, retroperitoneal videoassisted approaches have been developed. Necrotic tissue may be approached directly with a retroperitoneoscope or by intraoperative dilation of a drain tract, previously placed under CT guidance. In 1998 Gambiez et al. [50] first described the results of necrosectomy performed through a small (6 cm) left flank incision under visualization with a mediastinoscope in a series of 20 patients. Alternatively Carter [51] reported the use of a sinus tract endoscopy, which obviated the need for an incision. In this technique a percutaneous catheter drain tract is serially dilated to 30F under fluoroscopic guidance in the operating room and necrosectomy is performed under continuous irrigation using a nephroscope and a long grasping forceps in a piecemeal fashion. Connor et al. [52] applied the same technique in a series of 24 patients and reported a median of 3–4 procedures to completely remove all infected necrosis. Notably, this approach has the great advantage of avoiding peritoneal contamination, but it is limited in necrosis extraction, and the need for repeated sessions is quite common.

To obviate these limitations, in 2001 Horvath et al. [53] described a videoscopic assisted retroperitoneal debridement (VARD), in which a small (5 cm) subcostal flank incision was made to access the retroperitoneal space through which a videoscope was inserted via a single laparoscopic port. Debridement was performed through hydro-dissection and with the aid of long laparoscopic forceps inserted through a second port. In VARD, the small incision enables the surgeon to remove larger pieces of necrosis, with a shorter operating time and less need for repeat procedures. Complete necrosectomy, though, is not the ultimate aim of this procedure; only loosely adherent pieces of necrosis are removed, thereby keeping the risk of tearing underlying blood vessels to a minimum [54].

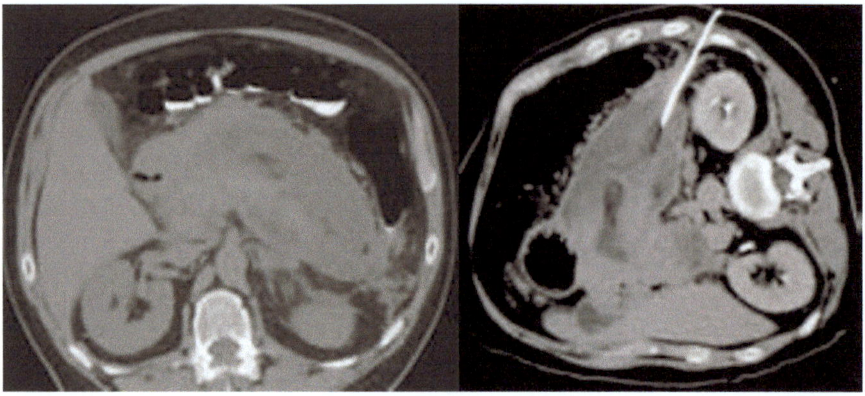

Fig. 4.1 This is the first step of a minimally invasive treatment of infected pancreatic necrosis: a CT-guided percutaneous drainage of pancreatic necrosis. This procedure should be performed through a retroperitoneal approach to allow a subsequent VARD when necessary

The results of this minimally invasive approach were recently published in two prospective studies, one single-arm [55] and one randomized [56]. When pancreatic necrosis required treatment as first step they used percutaneous or endoscopic drainage to mitigate sepsis (Fig. 4.1), in order to postpone or even obviate surgical necrosectomy. If drainage did not lead to clinical improvement, the percutaneous drain was used as a 'guidance drain' for VARD. Open surgery was left as the last step, to be performed in case of failure of more conservative treatment. This strategy, when compared to open surgery as first step, has been associated with a significantly lower morbidity (diabetes, incisional hernias and need of pancreatic enzyme) and lower new-onset multiple organ failure [56].

At present, none of the available guidelines provide precise recommendations for the use of minimally invasive techniques in clinical practice, but recent published guidelines (such as the Italian ones) suggest considering a less invasive approach than open surgery: *the presence of well-demarcated necrosis could be treated using percutaneous drainage; in selected cases, this approach can be combined with a minimally invasive surgical approach (videoscopic assisted retroperitoneal debridement)* [8].

Following the results of the recent prospective studies with high level of evidence, the authors' opinion is that the step-up approach will become the next gold standard when pancreatic necrosis requires treatment. Open surgery should be reserved to patients who fail to respond to minimally invasive treatment.

4.2.3 Abdominal Compartment Syndrome

For patients with SAP, this is the only actual indication for surgery in the first days after onset. ACS is a clinical condition consisting of intra-abdominal hypertension and organ dysfunction [57]. It occurs early in the course of SAP and is estimated to affect around 30% of patients admitted to the intensive care unit [58]. Recent studies report a 50–75% mortality rate in patients who develop ACS, but it is not clear how interventions may have played a role in determining the outcome [58]. Management of ACS in severe acute pancreatitis requires conservative treatment such as avoiding excess fluid intake, and using bowel decompression techniques to reduce intra-abdominal volume, but in most patients surgical decompression is needed. Usually a midline laparostomy is performed; alternatively a bilateral subcostal approach may be used. The treatment leads to reduction of intra-abdominal pressure, but there is still no evidence that this technique impacts on patient outcome.

4.3 Conclusions

In gallstone pancreatitis, laparoscopic cholecystectomy is indicated to prevent disease recurrence. In mild pancreatitis, it should be performed during the same hospital admission, as soon as the patient has recovered.

In case of severe pancreatitis, when pancreatic necrosis requires treatment, a minimally invasive approach should be considered whenever possible. The first step should be percutaneous drainage, followed, if necessary, by minimal invasive retroperitoneal debridement, with open surgery being reserved for patients who fail to respond to more conservative treatments.

References

1. Yadav D, Lowenfels AB (2006) Trends in the epidemiology of the first attack of acute pancreatitis: a systematic review. Pancreas 33:323-330
2. Frey CF, Zhou H, Harvey DJ, White RH (2006) The incidence and case-fatality rates of acute biliary, alcoholic, and idiopathic pancreatitis in California, 1994-2001. Pancreas 33:336-344
3. Everhart JE, Ruhl CE (2009) Burden of digestive diseases in the United States. Part III: liver, biliary tract, and pancreas. Gastroenterology 136:1134-1144
4. Lund H, Tonnesen H, Tonnesen MH, Olsen O (2006) Long-term recurrence and death rates after acute pancreatitis. Scand J Gastroenterol 41:234-238
5. Bradley EL 3rd (1993) A clinically based classification system for acute pancreatitis. Summary of the International Symposium on Acute Pancreatitis, Atlanta, Ga, September 13 1992. Arch Surg 128: 586-590
6. Uomo G, Pezzilli R, Gabbrielli A et al (2007) Diagnostic assessment and outcome of acute pancreatitis in Italy: results of a prospective multicentre study. Dig Liver Dis 39:829-837
7. Balthazar EJ (2002) Acute pancreatitis: assessment of severity with clinical and CT evaluation. Radiology 223:603-613
8. Pezzilli R, Zerbi A, Di Carlo V et al (2010) Working Group of the Italian Association for the Study of the Pancreas on Acute Pancreatitis (2010). Practical guidelines for acute pancreatitis. Pancreatology10:523-535
9. Working Party of the British Society of Gastroenterology; Association of Surgeons of Great Britain and Ireland; Pancreatic Society of Great Britain and Ireland; Association of Upper GI Surgeons of Great Britain and Ireland (2005) UK guidelines for the management of acute pancreatitis. Gut 54:1-9

10. Sauerland S, Agresta F, Bergamaschi R et al (2006) Laparoscopy for abdominal emergencies: evidence-based guidelines of the European Association for Endoscopic Surgery. Surg Endosc 20:14-29
11. Aboulian A, Chan T, Yaghoubian A et al (2010) Early cholecystectomy safely decreases hospital stay in patients with mild gallstone pancreatitis: a randomized prospective study. Ann Surg 251:615-619
12. Sinha R (2008) Early laparoscopic cholecystectomy in acute biliary pancreatitis: the optimal choice? HPB (Oxford) 10:332-335
13. Nebiker CA, Frey DM, Hamel CT et al (2009) Early versus delayed cholecystectomy in patients with biliary acute pancreatitis. Surgery 145:260-264
14. De Rai P, Zerbi A, Castoldi L et al (2010) Surgical management of acute pancreatitis in Italy: lessons from a prospective multicentre study. HPB 12:597-604
15. Petrov MS, Savides TJ (2009) Systematic review of endoscopic ultrasonography versus endoscopic retrograde cholangiopancreatography for suspected choledocholithiasis. Br J Surg 96:967-974
16. Acosta JM, Katkhouda N, Debian KA et al (2006) Early ductal decompression versus conservative management for gallstone pancreatitis with ampullary obstruction: a prospective randomized clinical trial. Ann Surg 243:33-40
17. Ayub K, Imada R, Slavin J (2010). Endoscopic retrograde cholangiopancreatography in gallstone-associated acute pancreatitis. Cochrane Database Syst Rev 1:CD003630
18. Rogers SJ, Cello JP, Horn JK et al (2010) Prospective randomized trial of LC+LCBDE vs ERCP/S+LC for common bile duct stone disease. Arch Surg 145:28-33
19. Clayton ES, Connor S, Alexakis N, Leandros E (2006) Meta-analysis of endoscopy and surgery versus surgery alone for common bile duct stones with the gallbladder in situ. Br J Surg 93:1185-1191
20. Martin DJ, Vernon DR, Toouli J (2006) Surgical versus endoscopic treatment of bile duct stones. Cochrane Database Syst Rev 2:CD003327
21. Uhl W, Warshaw A, Imrie C et al (2002) International Association of Pancreatology: IAP guidelines for the surgical management of acute pancreatitis. Pancreatology 2:565-573
22. Kelly TR, Wagner DS (1988). Gallstone pancreatitis: a prospective randomized trial of the timing of surgery. Surgery 104:600-605
23. Petrov MS, van Santvoort HC, Besselink MG et al (2008) Early endoscopic retrograde cholangiopancreatography versus conservative management in acute biliary pancreatitis without cholangitis: a meta-analysis of randomized trials. Ann Surg 247:250-257
24. Banks PA, Freeman ML, and the Practice Parameters Committee of the American College of Gastroenterology (2006) Practice guidelines in acute pancreatitis. Am J Gastroenterol 101:2379-2400
25. van Santvoort HC, Besselink MG, de Vries AC et al (2009) Early endoscopic retrograde cholangiopancreatography in predicted severe acute biliary pancreatitis: a prospective multicenter study. Ann Surg 250:68-75
26. Büchler MW, Gloor B, Müller CA et al (2000) Acute necrotizing pancreatitis: treatment strategy according to the status of infection. Ann Surg 232:619-626
27. Besselink MG, van Santvoort HC, Boermeester MA et al (2009) Timing and impact of infections in acute pancreatitis. Br J Surg 96:267-273
28. Banks P, Gerzof S, Langevin R et al (2005) CT-guided aspiration of suspected pancreatic infection: bacteriology and clinical outcome. Int J Pancreatol 18:265-270
29. Bradley EL 3rd, Allen K (1991) A prospective longitudinal study of observation versus surgical intervention in the management of necrotizing pancreatitis. Am J Surg 161:19-24
30. Mier J, Luque-de León E, Castillo A et al (1997) Early versus late necrosectomy in severe necrotizing pancreatitis. Am J Surg 173:71-75
31. Besselink MG, Verwer TJ, Schoenmaeckers EJ et al (2007) Timing of surgical intervention in necrotizing pancreatitis. Arch Surg 142:1194-1201
32. Fernandez-del Castillo C, Rattner DW, Makary MA et al (1998) Debridement and closed packing for the treatment of necrotizing pancreatitis. Ann Surg 228:676-684

33. Bradley EL III, Fulenwider JT (1984) Open treatment of pancreatic abscess. Surg Gynecol Obstet 159:509-513
34. Rodriguez JR, Razo AO, Targarona J et al (2008) Debridement and closed packing for sterile or infected necrotizing pancreatitis: insights into indications and outcomes in 167 patients. Ann Surg 247:294-299
35. Connor S, Alexakis N, Raraty MG et al (2005) Early and late complications after pancreatic necrosectomy. Surgery 137:499-505
36. Tsiotos GG, Luque-de León E, Sarr MG (1998) Long-term outcome of necrotizing pancreatitis treated by necrosectomy. Br J Surg 85:1650-1653
37. Howard TJ, Patel JB, Zyromski N et al (2007) Declining morbidity and mortality rates in the surgical management of pancreatic necrosis. J Gastrointest Surg 11:43-49
38. Werner J, Feuerbach S, Uhl W et al (2005) Management of acute pancreatitis: from surgery to interventional intensive care. Gut 54:426-436
39. Jacobi CA, Zieren HU, Sabat R et al (1997) Local and systemic inflammation after laparotomy versus laparoscopy in a sepsis model in rats. Langenbecks Archiv Chirurgie 382[Suppl 1]:9-13
40. Freeny P, Houptmann E, Althaus S et al (1998) Percutaneous CT-guided catheter drainage of infected acute necrotizing pancreatitis: techniques and results. Am J Roentgenol 170:969-975
41. Echenique AM, Sleeman D, Yrizarry J et al (1998) Percutaneous catheter directed debridement of infected pancreatic necrosis: results in 20 patients. J Vasc Interv Radiol 9:565-571
42. Papachristou GI, Takahashi N, Chahal P et al (2007) Per oral endoscopic drainage/debridement of walled-off pancreatic necrosis. Ann Surg 245:943-951
43. Gardner TB, Chahal P, Papachristou GI et al (2009) A comparison of direct endoscopic necrosectomy with transmural endoscopic drainage for the treatment of walled off pancreatic necrosis. Gastrointest Endosc 69:1085-1094
44. Navaneethan U, Vege SS, Chari ST, Baron TH (2009) Minimally invasive techniques in pancreatic necrosis. Pancreas 38:867-875
45. Gagner M (1996) Laparoscopic treatment of acute necrotizing pancreatitis. Semin Laparosc Surg 3:21-28
46. Zhu J, Fan X, Zhang X (2001) Laparoscopic treatment of severe acute pancreatitis. Surg Endosc 15:146-148
47. Parekh D (2006) Laparoscopic-assisted pancreatic necrosectomy: a new surgical option for treatment of severe necrotizing pancreatitis. Arch Surg 141:895-902
48. Cuschieri A (2002) Pancreatic necrosis: pathogenesis and endoscopic management. Semin Laparosc Surg 9:54-63
49. Bucher P, Pugin F, Morel P (2008) Minimally invasive necrosectomy for infected necrotizing pancreatitis. Pancreas 36:113-119
50. Gambiez LP, Denimal FA, Porte HL et al (1998) Retroperitoneal approach and endoscopic management of peripancreatic necrosis collections. Arch Surg 133:66-72
51. Carter R (2003) Management of infected necrosis secondary to acute pancreatitis: a balanced role for minimal access techniques. Pancreatology 3:133-138
52. Connor S, Ghaneh P, Raraty M et al (2003) Minimally invasive retroperitoneal pancreatic necrosectomy. Dig Surg 20:270-277
53. Horvath K, Koo L, Ali A et al (2001) Laparoscopic assisted percutaneous drainage of infected necrosis. Surg Endosc 15:677-682
54. Van Santvoort HC, Besselink MG, Horvath KD et al (2007) Videoscopic assisted retroperitoneal debridement in infected necrotizing pancreatitis. HPB (Oxford) 9:156-159
55. Horvath K, Freeny P, Escallon J et al (2010) Safety and efficacy of video-assisted retroperitoneal debridement for infected pancreatic collections: a multicenter, prospective, single-arm phase 2 study. Arch Surg 145:817-825
56. van Santvoort HC, Besselink MG, Bakker OJ et al (2010) A step-up approach or open necrosectomy for necrotizing pancreatitis. N Engl J Med 362:1491-1502
57. Cheatham ML, Malbrain ML, Kirkpatrick A et al (2007) Results from the International Conference of Experts on Intra-abdominal Hypertension and Abdominal Compartment Syndrome, II: recommendations. Intensive Care Med 33:951-962

58. McKay CJ, Evans S, Sinclair M et al (1999) High early mortality rate from acute pancreatitis in Scotland, 1984-1995. Br J Surg 86:1302-1305

Suggested Readings

Sauerland S, Agresta F, Bergamaschi R, Borzellino G, Budzynski A, Champault G, Fingerhut A, Isla A, Johansson M, Lundorff P (2006) Laparoscopy for abdominal emergencies. Evidence-based guidelines of the European Association for Endoscopic Surgery. Surg Endosc 20:14–29

Agresta F, Ansaloni L, Baiocchi L, Bergamini C, Campanile FB, Carlucci M, Cocorullo G, Corradi A, Franzato B, Lupo M, Mandalà V, Mirabella A, Pernazza G, Piccoli M, Staudacher C, Vettoretto N, Zago M, Lettieri E, Levati A, Pietrini D, Scaglione M, De Masi S, De Placido G, Francucci M, Rasi M, Scaramuzza G, Del Favero AL (2011) Consensus Development Conference of the Società Italiana Chirurgia Endoscopica e nuove tecnologie (SICE); Associazione Chirurghi Ospedalieri Italiani (ACOI); Società Italiana di Chirurgia (SIC); Società Italiana Chirurgia d'Urgenza e Trauma (SICUT), Società Italiana Chirurghi dell'Ospedalità Privata (SICOP) and the European Association for Endoscopic Surgery (EAES). In press

Acute Appendicitis 5

Antonino Mirabella, Nereo Vettoretto, Massimo Lupo,
Fausto Di Marco and Vincenzo Mandalà

5.1 Introduction

Acute appendicitis is the leading cause of emergency surgery (250,000 operations every year in the United States), accounting for approximately 10% of inpatient admissions, with an incidence of 1/500–600 inhabitants, most commonly occurring in individuals less than 30 years of age and females (1.3–1.6/1). At a distance of a century from the first appendectomy codified by McBurney [1], in 1977 the Dutch surgeon Hans de Kok [2] performed the first laparoscope assisted appendectomy. Nonetheless, the technique remained almost unknown due to the local diffusion of his paper, until Semm [3], a German gynecologist, published the first laparoscopic appendectomy (LA) five years later.

Since then, despite the rapid diffusion of mini-invasive surgery (laparoscopic cholecystectomy for example was executed only two years after LA, but became the gold standard for the NIH in 1992), the laparoscopic approach to appendicular disease is still debated.

An initial explanation for this can be found in the difficulty to shift from performing open appendectomy (OA), a procedure which is universally considered safe, effective and with low morbidity. Furthermore, the conventional *limitations* to the laparoscopic approach should not be underestimated, which include longer operative times and a greater burden for the organizational structure, and thus have slowed the diffusion of LA.

Systematic reviews on the topic including contributions from the Cochrane collaboration and clinical evidence studies published in the British Medical Journal state that only moderate to low quality evidence support the advantage

A. Mirabella (✉)
Department of General and Emergency Surgery
"Villa Sofia – Cervello" Hospital Trust
Palermo, Italy

V. Mandalà, *The Role of Laparoscopy in Emergency Abdominal Surgery*,

of laparoscopy in terms of lowering wound infections, reducing postoperative pain, length of hospital stay and time to return to work. This is counterbalanced by a higher rate of intra-abdominal abscesses, and a slightly but statistically significant longer operative time (14 min). Indeed, when comparing the pre-2000 to the post-2000 period, we can note an improvement in postoperative ileus and operative time, but still the rate of postoperative abdominal abscesses remains high. Differences in costs do not seem to be significant, unless the surgeon chooses to use hi-tech dissection instruments, disposable trocars or mechanical staplers routinely [4–7].

Only in recent years have several surgical centers come to use this approach more often than in the early days of laparoscopic appendectomy. Also in our experience over a period from 1999 to 2010 we report an increase in LA vs. OA. We also report an increase in LA in complex cases such as elderly or obese patients, as well as in cases when clinical and instrumental findings show a complicated acute appendicitis (perforated, gangrenous with local or general peritonitis).

5.2 Materials and Methods

We report our experience in the surgical management of acute appendicitis from January 1999 to December 2010.

For OA, we make a right para-rectal incision which varies from less than 2–3 cm to longer depending on patient build and the severity of clinical findings, such that a median laparotomy is performed where necessary when patient presents findings of peritonitis.

For LA, we usually use the standard three-trocar technique, as described by Novellino [8]. A 10 mm umbilical trocar is positioned for the camera (30°), a 5 mm trocar is placed in the left iliac fossa and another 5 mm trocar in a suprapubic site. This technique is the best way to meet the ergonomic needs of the surgeon and achieve triangulation of the optical and operative trocars which always represents the basis for a good laparoscopic operation (in Figures 5.1-5.3 the main steps of procedure). With the trocars in this position the appendix can be extracted under optical vision from the same optical trocar, when possible. In other conditions (large appendix, use of an endo-GIA to cut appendicular base, need for an endo-Catch to remove the appendix), we use a 10–12 mm trocar in the left iliac fossa instead of a 5 mm trocar. This trocar, when necessary, enables the camera position to be varied in the left iliac fossa (Figs. 5.4-5.8).

5.3 Results

We performed 697 total appendectomies, of which 333 (47.8%) were LA. Of these, 136 were males and 197 were females with a mean age of 22.8 years (range 8–76 years). A total of 109 (32.7% of LA) were emergent procedures

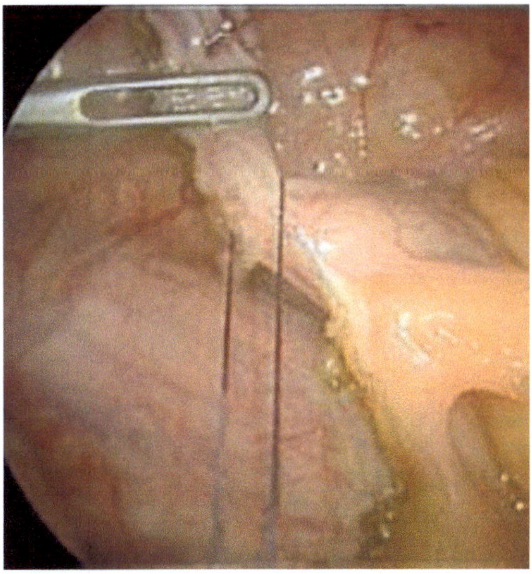

Fig. 5.1 Appendectomy begins with diathermy coagulation and dissection of the mesoappendix to the appendix down to its base. Once cleared to the cecum, the base of the appendix is ligated using one endoloop ligature

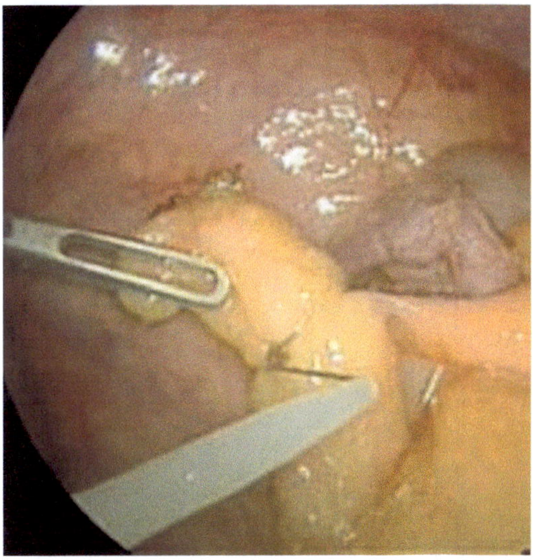

Fig. 5.2 Sometimes, after its dissection, the mesoappendix (with appendicular artery) can be secured by endoloop ligature (or haemostatic clip)

due to acute complicated appendicitis: 41 cases of gangrenous appendicitis, 25 perforated appendicitis, 43 local or diffuse peritonitis. Twenty-four out of 55 elderly patients (>65 years) underwent total LA (43.6%). Five of these (20.8%) had a complicated acute appendicitis. Forty-two LA were performed in obese patients (BMI >25).

The analysis of the eleven-year period shows an increase in the mini-invasive technique and a decrease in the traditional procedure (Fig. 5.9) Indeed in

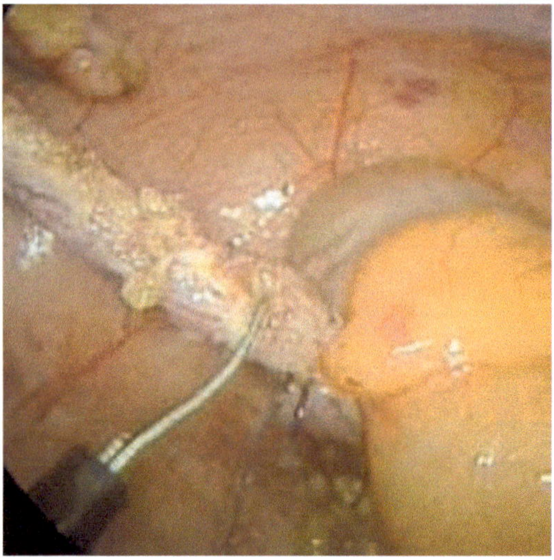

Fig. 5.3 The appendix is divided from the base and the mucosa is cauterized

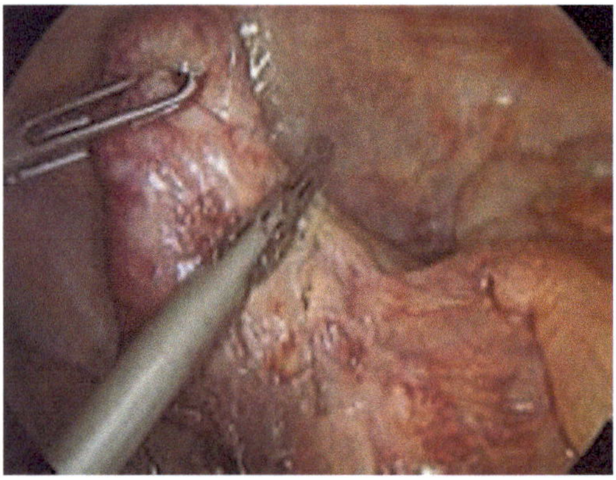

Fig. 5.4 A 32-year-old male patient. Abdominal pain in right iliac fossa and fever. Diagnostic laparoscopy: phlegmonous appendicitis. Skeletonization of the meso-appendix with ultrasonic dissector (ACE ETHICON)

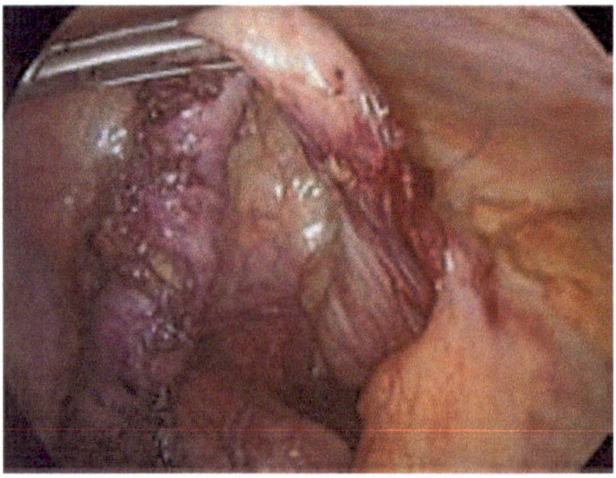

Fig. 5.5 Complete dissection to the base of cecal appendix

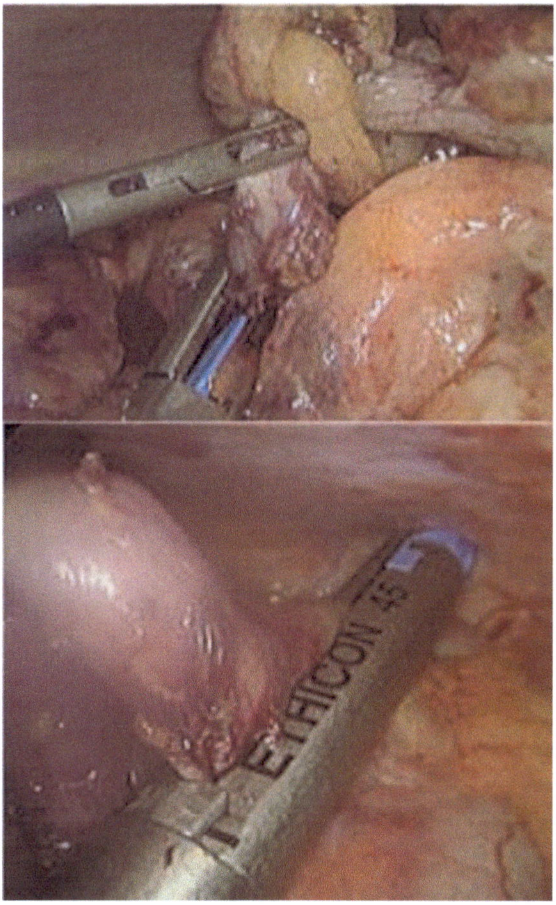

Fig. 5.6 Appendix section at the base with endo-GIA

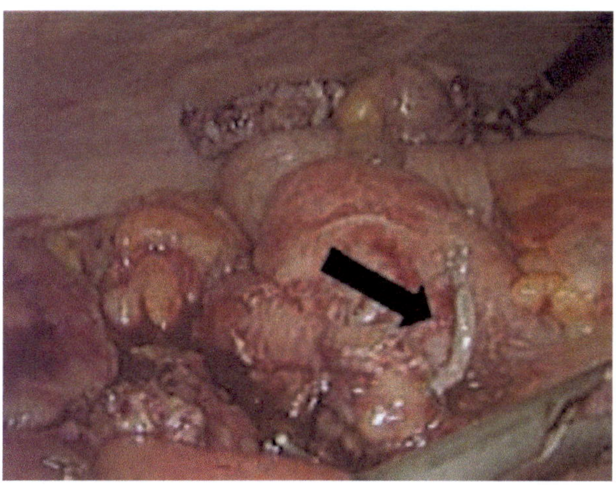

Fig. 5.7 Cecal appendicular stump

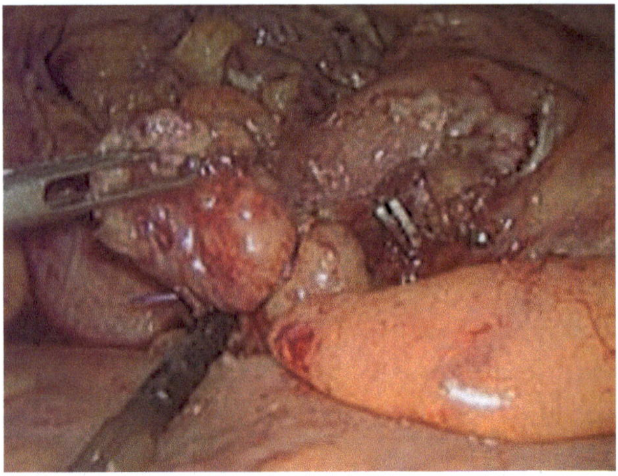

Fig. 5.8 Hemostasis of the appendicular mesentery is completed with endoloop (ETHICON Endo-suture system)

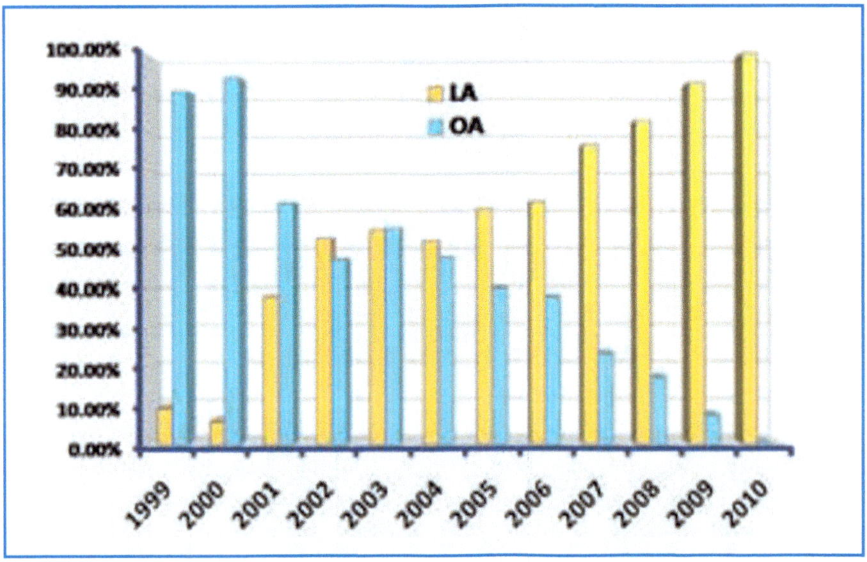

Fig. 5.9 Surgical management of all acute appendicitis from Jan 1999 to Dec 2010. *LA*, Laparoscopic Appendectomy; *OA*, Open Appendectomy

2010 a total of 100% of appendectomies were LA, even in the presence of complicated acute appendicitis (Fig. 5.10).

The average operative time was 64 min and ranged from 25 to 110 min. The operative time for LA was longer than OA but decreased progressively in later years thanks to increased skill of the surgical team (surgeons, anesthetist, OR nurses).

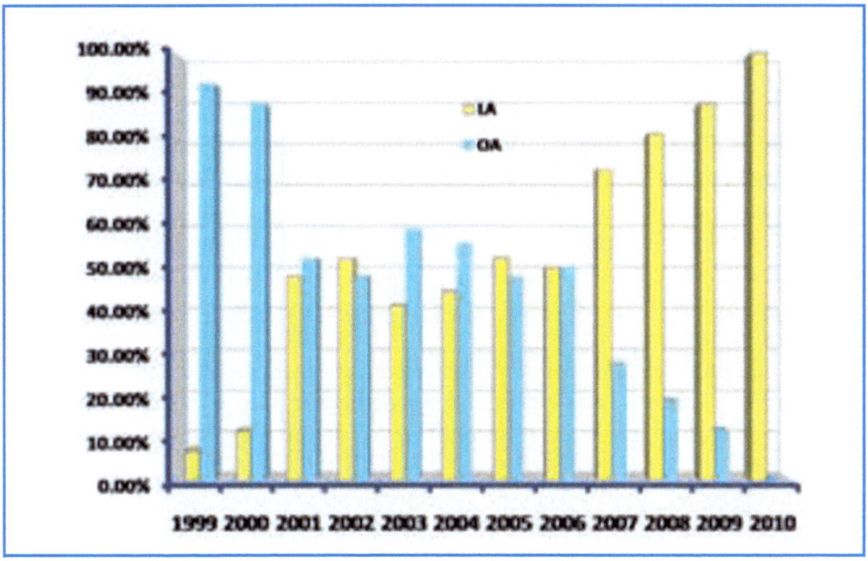

Fig. 5.10 Surgical management of acute complicated appendicitis from Jan 1999 to Dec 2010. *LA*, Laparoscopic Appendectomy; *OA*, Open Appendectomy

No significant differences between the two procedures in terms of postoperative hospital stay, oral intake and postoperative pain are reported.

The same data instead showed a better performance in terms of a diagnosis of complicated acute appendicitis in obese patients (when matched with larger laparotomies than McBurney incision) and in elderly patients in whom postoperative rehabilitation was more rapid.

In five patients a preoperative CT scan showed a pericecal suppurative mass likely from an acute perforated appendicitis. Two of these were treated by drainage, one percutaneous US-guided and one laparoscopic after failure of the US-guided percutaneous attempt. In the latter case the laparoscopic approach was unable to identify the appendix due to a serious intra-abdominal inflammatory condition and to an extensive pattern of pericecal adhesions with reduced work space. Drainage was removed after the 7th and 9th post-procedure day, respectively, after a regular clinical outcome and after US and CT controls. Interval appendectomy was planned after a strictly clinical and instrumental follow-up, but patients denied consent to the operation due to optimal clinical conditions. Follow-up at 12 and 36 months showed complete recovery.

One patient went into clinical remission after 24 hours of medical therapy and refused surgery, so continued antibiotic and infusive treatment under clinical, laboratory (WB, CRP), US and CT controls. Currently, at 13 months from clinical presentation, the patient is totally asymptomatic, and this condition has been confirmed by instrumental examinations.

One patient with a suppurative collection of the right psoas muscle was treated with medical therapy (antibiotic and infusive treatment) with remission of symptoms and CT evidence of a resolved suppurative collection. About 3 months later he suffered from abdominal pain and fever and underwent laparoscopic interval appendectomy with drainage of the residual collection.

The last patient of this series underwent drainage after an emergent xipho-pubic laparotomy. About 20 days later, abdominal pain, with fever, leukocytosis and CT finding of suppurative collection in the right iliac fossa prompted a re operation. An interval LA with drainage of residual suppurative collection was performed with success and the patient was discharged after 6 days from the repeat procedure.

In a patient that underwent LA, histologic findings showed a mucinous cistoadenoma. There was no evidence of appendicular perforation and the resection margin was intact. After 36 months of follow-up there was no evidence of recurrence.

Eight patients (2.4%) had major complications after LA: four cases of abdominal collection, one case of hemoperitoneum, two cases of bowel perforations and one leakage from the appendicular stump.

Hemorrhagic complications occurred in one 26-year-old patient 12 hours after LA due to acute catarrhal appendicitis. A repeat procedure was performed and about 1000 mL of blood was evacuated from the abdomen due to left epigastric vessel lesion. Hemostasis was performed by two trans-parietal sutures at the trocar site. The patient had a good outcome and was discharged after four days.

Of four patients with post-LA abscess (all operated for complicated acute appendicitis), two underwent laparoscopic evacuation of the collection (one pericecal and one located in the pelvis); one case of a small pericecal collection was resolved with antibiotic therapy; the 4th patient underwent laparotomic drainage after 3 weeks from LA. All cases had complete recovery.

In two patients who had undergone previous laparotomies, the insertion of the optic trocar by open technique at the site of umbilical scar caused a bowel loop lesion due to the massive adherence of the bowel loops with the previous laparotomic scar. In one patient the lesion was recognized and treated during LA. In the other the lesion went unrecognized and in the early postoperative period caused a periumbilical collection, as the abdominal CT showed, with clinical evidence of a low-flow enterocutaneous fistula on the umbilical scar, fever, leukocytosis and no bowel viability. Earlier laparotomy (2nd postoperative day) with direct suture of the bowel lesion solved the problem with a good patient outcome.

One patient with a leakage from the appendicular stump (histologic finding of appendix showed suspected Crohn disease) was successfully treated with medical therapy alone (antibiotic and infusive treatment).

Minor complications occurred in 11 patients: three trocar site incisional hernias and eight umbilical trocar site infections (respectively in two and four obese patients).

The conversion rate was 3.6% (12 patients), and was particularly high in complicated acute appendicitis (4.6% – five patients). This elevated the mean hospital stay (about 7 days), with a negative effect on postoperative outcomes (pain, oral intake, and return to job) and with an increase in parietal complications (scar infection in obese patient).

The causes of conversion were anatomical (no recognized appendix, bowel adhesions, extensive acute inflammation due to complicated appendicitis) and in one case an unforeseen perforated sigmoid diverticulum.

5.4 Discussion

Even though the laparoscopic approach has in recent times become widely used in several fields of abdominal surgery, it cannot be stated that LA is currently widely accepted as the approach of choice for acute appendicitis in preference to the traditional operation by all surgeons.

A survey carried out by ACOI in Italy in 2009 [7] regarding the diffusion of LA shows that only 23% of surgical divisions widely perform LA (>90% operated patients); 22% of surgical centers perform LA between 50 and 90% of cases; 48% of centers use LA for <50% of cases and another 7% never use LA. Only 48% of the surveyed centers make wide use of LA regardless of the type of patient or the presence of acute appendicitis.

This technique has several limitations: longer operative times, greater engagement of the organization (it requires a skilled surgical team – surgeons, nurses, anesthetist – especially in emergent procedures and at night), higher costs (due to longer operative times and for the technology of materials needed for the operation). Furthermore, although there is a significant number of studies in the literature which compare the two procedures (OA vs. LA) (thousands of indexed papers, many randomized studies, a number of meta-analyses, several case-control studies, retrospective studies and reviews), in contrast to other fields of laparoscopic surgery these studies are of limited use. They report discordant data, in part due to the poor quality of the methodological and statistic criteria used [9].

Despite the lack of significant, evidence-based advantages in the general comparison with OA, LA has become widespread in recent years, probably due to the increasing acquaintance with laparoscopy in other fields, in most surgical practices, in teaching hospitals as well as in district hospitals.

In our experience too, at the beginning, the technique was used for the learning curve of the surgeon in laparoscopic surgery training, but now we can say that we use the mini-invasive technique in all cases, even in complicated acute appendicitis, except when laparoscopy is generally contraindicated.

With the passing of time, thanks to better work organization (better skill of surgical teams in emergent laparoscopic procedures performed right around the clock, shorter operative times and lower costs of laparoscopic materials) and moreover thanks to of the large number of procedures performed over these years, the drawbacks of LA have been minimized and the advantages have been enhanced, such as better diagnostic accuracy with complete exploration of the abdominal cavity, diagnosis and treatment of associated diseases, better postoperative performance, lower morbidity, better comfort of the patients and shorter hospital stay. This is especially true for women in premenopausal age, in whom there is solid evidence of the advantages of laparoscopy. As for cases of complicated acute appendicitis and obese patients, in whom the alternative is not a small incision in the right iliac fossa, but rather a large and destructive laparotomy, the advantages are evident to those practicing LA, although they are not supported by evidence. In fact, the demonstrated reduction of wound and pulmonary infections is counterbalanced by a higher rate of intra-abdominal abscesses, and as reported in some recent RCTs by higher costs when compared to open access [10, 11].

A correct diagnosis of acute appendicitis is based on a thorough history and clinical examination (in the case of reproductive-age women a gynecologic examination is useful) and on laboratory work-up (WBC and serum CRP [12]) and on some instrumental examinations (first-line abdominal US [13] and second-line abdominal CT scan [14]).

The use of the mini-invasive technique, i.e. always a surgical technique that requires general anesthesia, is justified for diagnostic purposes only when there is a strong diagnostic doubt. We can consider two clinical patterns:

- clinical evidence of acute appendicitis with positive laboratory tests and positive US examination: emergent laparoscopic appendectomy. Particular attention should be paid to elderly patients in whom there is a high risk of perforation. In these cases an emergent abdominal CT examination is useful and surgery should be performed as soon as possible;
- in those atypical clinical cases and/or when laboratory tests and US fails to confirm clinical suspicion, we retain that *active observation* (AO) [15] is the best way to reach a diagnosis. This consists of close follow-up of the patient with clinical and instrumental controls (every few hours), gynecologic examination for young reproductive-age women in whom gynecologic disease could mimic an acute appendicitis, while an abdominal CT scan would be considered a second-line examination. However, when AO proves unable to clarify the clinical pattern, especially in female patients, a diagnostic laparoscopy may be indicated.

Our experience over recent years and the results we have obtained have convinced us to always perform LA except when the mini-invasive approach is impossible due to general contraindications. Therefore, we have broadened the use of mini-invasive surgery not only to patients with typical indications (reproductive-age women, doubt and prolonged AO), but also to the elderly, obese subjects, and cases of complicated acute appendicitis (gangrenous appendicitis, perforated appendicitis, local or generalized peritonitis).

Some of the advantages in young patients can also be found in the elderly with acute appendicitis, although reaching a correct diagnosis is crucial given the high risk of complicated forms.

In our small clinical series (LA in 24 patients >65 years – five with complicated forms) we obtained good results in line with those in the literature [16, 17], especially in terms of a quicker return to normal activities than in OA, particularly in the complicated forms (three gangrenous, one perforated and one pelviperitonitis).

The advantages of laparoscopic surgery in obese patients have been amply described. These include better exploration of the abdominal cavity and less parietal injury than in larger laparotomies. The advantages of the laparoscopic technique are particularly notable in obese patients: less postoperative pain, less parietal septic complications, less incidence of incisional hernias, less adhesive syndrome [11]. These advantages seem more evident in obese patients particularly when the appendicitis is complicated, given the lower incidence of complications (from 27% to 18%) and lower costs than open surgery in obese patients with a diagnosis of perforated appendicitis [18].

In our experience overall parietal morbidity was 14.2% in 42 obese patients who underwent LA (two incisional trocar site hernias, two hematomas, four trocar site infections).

This morbidity was lower than in OA, which was 32% in 156 patients (24 suppurations, 10 hematomas/seromas of the scar and 16 incisional hernias). All of these had a larger laparotomy than McBurney's incision.

The rate of parietal infections in the obese patients was 9.5% (4 cases) in LA vs. 15.3% (24 cases) in OA.

Currently the use of LA in acute complicated appendicitis is debated. Several authors report a greater number of visceral lesions and particularly related to intra-abdominal abscess in LA than in OA [19–21], so these authors advise against the mini-invasive technique in complicated acute appendicitis.

In our reports there was an overall rate of intra-abdominal abscess of 1.4% after LA (4 patients). This figure increases to 4.2% in cases of LA for complicated appendicitis, whereas the rate of parietal infections was 2.8% (8 patients). These figures are similar to those of Cochrane Database of Systematic Reviews [22].

This large database from a review of 54 controlled randomized trials, with about 5000 patients, shows an intra-abdominal infection rate of 0.6% in OA and of 1.8% after LA. However, parietal infection is higher in OA than LA – 7.6% vs. 3.8%.

These results have been criticized for the quality of the studies and have not been confirmed by the experiences of other authors. In fact in their opinion the problem of intra-abdominal abscess post-LA is lower [23].

Given their experience, they consider the technique to be safe and useful even in more complex situations, where laparoscopy is unable to offer reduced parietal damage or a complete exploration of the abdominal cavity and extensive lavage of the peritoneal recesses [24, 25]. Indeed, peritoneal lavage is scarcely standardized in the literature. Apart from a retrospective paper that suggests extensive lavage as a possible cause of contamination and postoperative abscesses, there is an experimental study that relies on at least 6 L of lavage to lower the bacterial concentration in children with appendicitis [26, 27]. Particularly in these circumstances the surgeon's skill and a well codified technique are fundamental for achieving an optimal result and for reducing the overall complication rate and the overall conversion rate to open surgery. The decision to convert a LA in an open procedure is a delicate choice that should be taken with great care. In fact, although it is often a mandatory choice for patient safety, it is also true that it can have negative consequences on postoperative outcomes (overall hospital stay, postoperative pain, oral intake and return to work) and on parietal complications (increased risk of infection of the laparotomic scar).

More frequent causes of mandatory conversion include anatomic conditions, especially in complicated cases, such as reduced abdominal working space, failure to identify the appendix and dense visceral adhesions.

The number of laparoscopic procedures performed by a surgeon over the years seems to play a decisive role in the frequency of conversion, as shown by Hellberg et al. [28], who report an extremely varied rate of conversion (from 17% to 71%) related to the surgeon's level of experience. Our overall conversion rate after LA for total procedures (3.6% – 12 patients) and after LA in complicated appendicitis (4.6% – 5 patients) relates to the early years of our experience (the last case in 2005). This seems to confirm that conversion is strictly related not only to the severity of the clinical and anatomopathologic pattern, but also to experience acquired by the surgeon in laparoscopic surgery.

A particular case is the treatment of appendicular mucocele. The type of procedure to be performed is a matter of debate: a simple appendectomy (laparoscopic, after immediate conversion or if open appendectomy is mandatory?) in initial forms, or a large colic resection, associated with complementary therapies (hyperthermic intraperitoneal chemotherapy, peritonectomy, post operative chemotherapy) in advanced phases, as proposed by Dhage-Ivatury and Sugarbaker [29].

In our experience only one patient with initial phase mucocele was treated with LA associated with a large resection of the cecal cap by endo-GIA stapler. In this case, we think that the uninjured resection margins of the specimen with no perforation signs (*benign mucocele*) and a gentle manipulation of the appendix enabled mini-invasive treatment to be performed safely enough to avoid the possible iatrogenic spread of the disease to the peritoneum (*pseudomyxoma peritonei*) [29, 30].

Five patients with a peri-appendicular abscess underwent conservative treatment (simple drainage of the collection without appendectomy): one US-guided abdominal drainage; one laparoscopic abdominal drainage; two cases of antibiotic therapy and clinical-instrumental follow-up and one emergent umbilical-pubic laparotomy and peri-collection drainage.

We obtained complete remission of the clinical condition in three patients and appendectomy was not necessary. In two patients (one underwent laparotomy and drainage; one was treated with medical therapy) a laparoscopic interval appendectomy with drainage of the residual collection was necessary due to a recurrence of symptoms and an increase in the residual collection seen at abdominal CT.

Currently there is no global consensus as to whether this treatment is correct because many questions remain unanswered, such as the risk of recurrence of the collection, the incidence of complications, potentially underestimated neoplastic lesions and the indication and timing for definitive treatment [31–34]. However, we agree with Meshikhes [35], who considers conservative treatment a possible alternative to emergent appendectomy in the presence of an *appendicular mass*.

Interval appendectomy could prove useful, especially in children, but generally not as definitive treatment. The indications and timing of the procedure would need to be evaluated on the basis of clinical and instrumental findings. A recent systematic review concerning conservative treatment versus early appendectomy in patients with inflammatory appendicular masses seems to reserve a role for interval appendectomy also in the adult setting [36].

Another question is whether increased use of the mini-invasive technique would modify the approach to a patient with a possible appendicular colic, thus reducing the number of false positives and therefore the number of useless appendectomies. There is no clear answer because the decision taken can vary from one surgeon to the next in the presence of a macroscopically healthy appendix. In fact more often than not an appendectomy is performed instead of leaving the healthy appendix in situ.

As in the open technique, we too have always performed an appendectomy after previous explorative laparoscopy. There are some justifications for this behavior: the risk of a false negative at the anatomopathologic examination of the appendix (up to 26% of *endoappendicitis* [37]), and no increased morbidity and no increased postoperative hospital stay with respect to diagnostic laparoscopy [38]. A recent case series shows that a particular benefit (in terms of recurrent symptoms) might be found for those patients affected by fecoliths, which might cause appendicular colicky pain [39].

In contrast to this treatment approach other surgeons prefer a conservative approach because the incidence of acute appendicitis after diagnostic laparoscopy and conservation of the appendix is the same as control cases [40]. A recent clinical evidence review reports up to 12% of emergent surgery and 35% of appendectomies in the following year in those treated conservatively [5].

However, a conservative approach may be applied in the presence of a healthy appendix when others intra-abdominal conditions (gynecologic disease) can justify the symptoms.

5.5 Conclusions

The choice of preferring LA seems to be justified for several reasons:

- better diagnostic accuracy thanks to complete abdominal exploration;

- diagnosis and treatment of possible associated diseases (particularly gynecologic diseases);
- better postoperative performance (lower morbidity, less discomfort and shorter hospital stay).

The advantages of mini-invasive surgery are more evident in obese patients or in the presence of complicated appendicitis, when the alternative to LA is not a small incision at the right iliac fossa, but a wide median laparotomy.

From our experience and from the literature we can draw the following conclusions.

The use of diagnostic laparoscopy is recommended only in selected cases, when diagnostic doubt remains even after thorough clinical and instrumental observation (*active observation*) or when there is persistence or a worsening of the symptoms. This is particularly true in young reproductive-age women, where the laparoscopic technique could be an aid in the differential diagnosis with gynecologic disease.

LA may be performed in all patients except when general or local conditions contraindicate LA. Therefore, LA is indicated not only for young reproductive-age women and patients with a diagnostic doubt, but also for other groups traditionally considered not able to undergo laparoscopy such as the elderly, obese patients and cases of complicated appendicitis.

Of course, in cases of complicated acute appendicitis LA is a more complex procedure, with a higher complication rate and higher conversion rate. It has been shown that in these cases the surgeon's experience and the use of a standardized technique are the best ways to obtain an optimal result.

Interval appendectomy can be a possible therapeutic option in cases of conservative treatment of *appendicular mass* and its indication and timing should be evaluated on clinical and instrumental findings.

Not so clear is the approach when the appendix is macroscopically healthy at laparoscopic exploration: always appendectomy or wait and see? We believe the first choice is justified by several considerations: no increase in postoperative morbidity; hospital stay no longer than simple diagnostic laparoscopy, risk of endoappendicitis; prophylactic appendectomy.

References

1. McBurney C (1889) Experience with early operative interference in cases of disease of the vermiform appendix. NY Med J 50:676-684
2. de Kok H (1977) A new technique for resecting the non-inflamed not-adhesive appendix through a mini-laparotomy with the aid of the laparoscope. Acta Chir Need 29:195-198
3. Semm K (1983) Endoscopic appendectomy. Endoscopy 15:59-64
4. Sauerland S, Jaschinski T, Neugebauer EA (2010) Laparoscopic versus open surgery for suspected appendicitis. Cochrane Database Syst Rev 10:CD001546
5. D'Souza N (2011) Appendicitis. Clin Evid 01:408
6. Gorenoi V, Dintsios CM, Schönermark M, Hagen A (2006) Laparoskopische vs. offene Appendektomie. Systematische Übersicht zur medizinischen Wirksamkeit und gesundheitsökonomische Analyse. HTA-Bericht 148. In: Deutsche Agentur für Health Technology As-

sessment des Deutschen Instituts für Medizinische Dokumentation und Information (DAHTA@DIMDI) (Hrsg.). Schriftenreihe Health Technology Assessment (HTA) in der Bundesrepublik Deutschland. DAHTA-Datenbank des DIMDI, Köln

7. Vettoretto N, Gobbi S, Belli F et al (2011) Diffusion of laparoscopic appendectomies in Italy: a National audit. Minim Invasive Ther Allied Technol [Epub ahead of print] doi: 10.3109/13645706.2011.557079
8. Novellino L (1996) Appendicectomia. Chirurgia laparoscopica: quaderni di tecnica (vol. II). Stampe grafiche Mariano
9. Kapischke M, Caliebe A, Tepel J et al (2006) Open versus laparoscopic appendectomy. Surg Endosc 20:1060-1068
10. Markides G, Subar D, Riyad K (2010) Laparoscopic versus open appendectomy in adults with complicated appendicitis: a systematic review and meta-analysis. World J Surg 34:2026-2040
11. Ricca R, Schneider JJ, Brar H, Lucha PA (2007) Laparoscopic appendectomy in patients with a body mass index of 25 or greater: results of a double blind, prospective, randomized trial. JSLS 11:54-58
12. Pruekprasert P, Maipang T, Geater A et al (2004) Accuracy in diagnosis of acute appendicitis by comparing serum C-reactive protein measurements, Alvarado score and clinical impression of surgeons. J Med Assoc Thai 87:296-303
13. Poortman P, Oostvogel HJ, Bosma E et al (2009) Improving diagnosis of acute appendicitis: results with standard use of ultrasonography followed by selective use of CT. J Am Surg 208:434-441
14. Rao PM, Rhea JT, Novelline RA et al (1998) Effect of computed tomography of the appendix on treatment of patients and use of hospital resources. N Engl J Med 338:141-146
15. Morino M, Pellegrino L, Castagna E (2006) Acute nonspecific abdominal pain. A randomized, controlled trial comparing early laaroscopy versus clinical observation. Ann Surg 244:881-888
16. Harrell AG, Lincourt AE, Novitsky YW et al (2006) Advantages of laparoscopic appendectomy in the elderly. Am Surg 72:474-480
17. Kirshtein B, Perry ZH, Mizrahi S, Lantsberg L (2009) Value of laparoscopic appendectomy in the elderly patient. World J Surg 33:918-922
18. Varela JE, Hinojosa MW, Nguyen NT (2008) Laparoscopy should be the approach of choice for acute appendicitis in the morbidly obese. Am J Surg 196:218-222
19. Pokala N, Sadhasivam S, Kiran RP, Parithivel V (2007) Complicated appendicitis - is the laparoscopic approach appropriate? A comparative study with the open approach: outcome in a community hospital setting. Am Surg 73:737-741
20. Paik PS, Towson JA, Anthone GJ (1997) Intra-abdominal abscesses following laparoscopic and open appendectomies. J Gastrointest Surg 1:188-193
21. Pedersen AG, Petersen OB, Wara P et al (2001) Randomized controlled trial of laparoscopic versus open appendectomy. Br J Surg 88:200-205
22. Sauerland S, Lefering R, Neugebauer EA (2004) Laparoscopic versus open surgery for suspected appendicitis. Cochrane Database Syst Rev 18:CD001546
23. Kouwenhoven EA, Repelaer van Driel OJ, van Erp WF (2005) Fear for the intraabdominal abscess after laparoscopic appendectomy: not realistic. Surg Endosc 19:923-926
24. Lin HF, Wu JM, Tseng LM et al (2006) Laparoscopic versus open appendectomy for perforated appendicitis. J Gastrointest Surg 10:906-910
25. Fukami Y, Hasegawa H, Sakamoto E et al (2007) Value of laparoscopic appendectomy in perforated appendicitis. World J Surg 31:93-97
26. Gupta G, Sample C, Bamehriz F, Birch DW (2006) Infectious complications following laparoscopic appendectomy. Can J Surg 49:397-400
27. Ohno Y, Furui J, Kanematsu T (2004) Treatment strategy when using intraoperative peritoneal lavage for perforated appendicitis in children: a preliminary report. Pediatr Surg Int 20:534-537
28. Hellberg A, Rudberg C, Enochsson L et al (2001) Conversion from laparoscopic to open appendicectomy: a possible drawback of the laparoscopic technique? Eur J Surg 167:209-213

29. Dhage-Ivatury S, Sugarbaker PH (2006) Update on the surgical approach to mucocele of the appendix. J Am Coll Surg 202:680-684
30. Karakaya K, Barut F, Emre AU et al (2008) Appendiceal mucocele: case reports and review of current literature. World J Gastroenterol 14:2280-2283
31. Corfield L (2007) Interval appendicectomy after appendiceal mass or abscess in adults: what is "best practice"? Surg Today 37:1-4
32. Tekin A, Kurtoglu HC, Can I, Oztan S (2008) Routine interval appendectomy is unnecessary after conservative treatment of appendiceal mass. Colerectal Dis 10:465-468
33. Lugo JZ, Avgerinos DV, Leftkowitz AJ et al (2010) Can interval appendectomy be justified following conservative treatment of perforated acute appendicitis? J Surg Res 164:91-94
34. Keckler SJ, Tsao K, Sharp SW et al (2008) Resource utilization and outcomes from percutaneous drainage and interval appendectomy for perforated appendicitis with abscess. J Pediatric Surg 43:977-980
35. Meshikhes AW (2008) Management of appendiceal mass: controversial issues revisited. J Gastrointest Surg 12:767-775
36. Simillis C, Symeonides P, Shorthouse AJ, Tekkis PP (2010) A meta-analysis comparing conservative treatment versus acute appendectomy for complicated appendicitis (abscess or phlegmon). Surgery 147:818-829
37. Kraemer M, Ohmann C, Leppert R, Yang Q (2000) Macroscopic assessment of the appendix at diagnostic laparoscopic is reliable. Surg Endosc 14:625-633
38. Greason KL, Rappold JF, Liberman MA (1998) Incidental laparoscopic appendectomy for acute right lower quadrant abdominal pain. Surg Endosc 12:223-225
39. Grimes C, Bailey C, Gergely S, Harris A (2010) Appendiceal faecaliths are associated with right iliac fossa pain. Ann R Coll Surg Engl 92:61-64
40. Van de Broek WT, Bijnen AB, de Ruiter P, Gouma DJ (2001) A normal appendix found during diagnostic laparoscopic should not be removed. Br J Surg 88:251-254

Suggested Readings

Sauerland S, Agresta F, Bergamaschi R, Borzellino G, Budzynski A, Champault G, Fingerhut A, Isla A, Johansson M, Lundorff P (2006) Laparoscopy for abdominal emergencies. Evidence-based guidelines of the European Association for Endoscopic Surgery. Surg Endosc 20:14–29

Agresta F, Ansaloni L, Baiocchi L, Bergamini C, Campanile FB, Carlucci M, Cocorullo G, Corradi A, Franzato B, Lupo M, Mandalà V, Mirabella A, Pernazza G, Piccoli M, Staudacher C, Vettoretto N, Zago M, Lettieri E, Levati A, Pietrini D, Scaglione M, De Masi S, De Placido G, Francucci M, Rasi M, Scaramuzza G, Del Favero AL (2011) Consensus Development Conference of the Società Italiana Chirurgia Endoscopica e nuove tecnologie (SICE); Associazione Chirurghi Ospedalieri Italiani (ACOI); Società Italiana di Chirurgia (SIC); Società Italiana Chirurgia d'Urgenza e Trauma (SICUT), Società Italiana Chirurghi dell'Ospedalità Privata (SICOP) and the European Association for Endoscopic Surgery (EAES). In press

Role of Laparoscopy in the Treatment of Acute Diverticulitis: an Evidence-Based Review

6

Boris Franzato, Stefano Mandalà, Grazia Fusco and Carlo Sartori

6.1 Introduction

The incidence of diverticular disease is rising, mainly among younger patients [1]. The severity of the disease ranges from light symptomatic diverticulosis to perforated diverticulitis. For years it was thought that the risk of perforation and other complications increased after each recurrence. Therefore, the European Association of Endoscopic Surgery (EAES) consensus conference of 1999 [2] suggested performing an elective sigmoid resection after two episodes of acute diverticulitis, after a single episode in young patients, in immunosuppressed patients or when complications such as stenosis or fistulae occur. However, new insights into the natural course of diverticular disease have resulted in a more conservative approach, which is the current trend. Severe complicated diverticulitis, leading to emergent surgical intervention, is most often the primary presentation of the disease [3]. Recent studies have shown that recurrent episodes of diverticulitis have a low complication rate in patients treated conservatively for an acute episode of diverticulitis [3, 4]. It seems that elective, prophylactic sigmoid resections based on the number of episodes are not always indicated. New diagnostic tools and therapeutic techniques have improved the treatment of diverticular disease. The possibility of treating abscesses by computed tomography (CT) and percutaneous drainage has shown that emergency surgery can in many cases be delayed and that an elective resection can be done when indicated [5]. The rise of laparoscopic surgery since the 1990s has resulted, alongside the general advantages of mini-invasive surgery, in decreased morbidity and mortality rates compared to open approaches, making it progressively the preferred approach in elective colonic resections [6].

B. Franzato (✉)
General Surgery, "San Giacomo Apostolo" Hospital,
Castelfranco Veneto (TV), Italy

V. Mandalà, *The Role of Laparoscopy in Emergency Abdominal Surgery*,

Whether laparoscopy can also be applied to patients with perforated diverticulitis and generalized peritonitis remains under debate. Laparoscopic sigmoid resection cannot always be accomplished completely because of extensive pericolic inflammation and fecal or purulent contamination, or due to patient conditions and comorbidity. Hartmann's procedure remains the treatment of first choice for most surgeons. However, several recent studies have shown that a primary anastomosis with or without a deviating ostomy could be performed safely even under these circumstances [4]. Laparoscopic lavage and drainage can be a safe alternative to Hartmann's procedure in cases of perforated purulent diverticulitis, if a laparoscopic approach is indicated [7].

We report the results obtained by a single institution, expert in laparoscopic surgery, with a literature review on actual trends of laparoscopic management in acute diverticular diseas,e and highlight levels of evidence for clinical practice.

6.2 Personal Experience

From August 1994 to September 2010 in the Surgical Department of San Giacomo Hospital in Castelfranco Veneto, Italy, 1,348 laparoscopic colectomies were performed. Of these, 286 were for diverticular disease. Hinchey IV patients were excluded because they were operated directly by laparotomy or converted.

All patients admitted for suspected diverticulitis underwent a CT scan with intravenous contrast. All the elective patients after diagnostic study were offered a minimally invasive operation. Urgent cases were managed laparoscopically unless the patient had refused laparoscopic surgery, was too hemodynamically unstable to tolerate a pneumoperitoneum or had cardiopulmonary comorbidity contraindicating a laparoscopic approach. The current study includes all the patients with primary diagnoses of diverticular disease including diverticulosis, acute diverticulitis, and chronic diverticulitis. Only patients undergoing laparoscopic operative management of diverticular disease were considered. All the patients underwent laparoscopic colectomy with unprotected primary anastomosis or laparoscopic lavage-drainage, at the surgeon's discretion. All colectomies were performed using straight laparoscopy. No hand-assist devices were used. In addition, ureteric stents were not used routinely.

The definition of complicated diverticular disease used in this series was modeled on the 1999 EAES Consensus Conference [2]. Complicated diverticular disease was thus defined as acute pericolic abscess (Hinchey 1), acute pelvic abscess (Hinchey 2), purulent peritonitis (Hinchey 3), fecal peritonitis (Hinchey 4), fistula, stricture, hemorrhage.

Uncomplicated cases were defined as simple diverticulitis refractory to medical management with important symptoms, recurrent or chronic diverticulitis, and noninflammatory complications of diverticulosis.

The patients consisted of 136 males and 150 females aged from 24 to 87 years (mean 62.5 years). A total of 55 patients (19.23%) were ≤50 years.

A total of 97 patients were classified ASA1 (33.92%), 159 ASA2 (55.59%) and 30 ASA3 (10.49%).

Indications for elective laparoscopic treatment were recurrent episodes of severe diverticulitis (two or more), with radiologic evidence of important colonic alterations (asymmetry, wall thickening, stenosis) and/or complications of the disease after initial conservative management.

Indications for urgent laparoscopic treatment were patients with CT and clinical evidence of peritonitis who were fit, stable and without signs of septic shock. Nine patients (3.14%) underwent urgent laparoscopic lavage and drainage for purulent peritonitis (Hinchey 3), five of whom were operated after 4–6 weeks with elective laparoscopic sigmoid resection and four sent for follow-up.

Our standardized operative technique and strategy in diverticulitis have been described elsewhere [8, 9].

6.3 Results

A total of 286 patients with diagnosis of diverticular disease were considered for analysis. Of these, 83 (29.02%) patients had complicated disease, whereas 203 (70.98%) patients had uncomplicated disease.

Thirty-five (12.24%) patients had pericolic abscess (Hinchey 1), seven (2.45%) pelvic abscess (Hinchey 2); 16 patients (5.59%) had a chronic diverticulitis complicated with stricture, eight with colovescical fistula (2.80%), four with colovaginal fistula (1.40%), two with ileocolic fistula (0.70%). Two patients (0.70%) had acute bleeding requiring preoperative emergency treatment by means of transfemoral embolization followed by elective laparoscopic colonic resection. Diverticula were mostly in the descending colon and sigmoid, in two cases we observed right-sided diverticula.

We performed 247 left colectomies, 28 sigmoidectomies, one subtotal colectomy, one ileocecal resection and nine procedures of laparoscopic lavage and drainage. In 15 patients an additional procedure was associated: six cholecystectomies, five adnexectomies, three appendectomies, one hysterectomy. All resected patients received an unprotected primary anastomosis except for four cases in which a protective ileostomy was performed.

Closed suction drainage was used only in particularly difficult cases or if there was any doubt about the quality of the anastomosis, in spite of negative air test. Mean operative time was 160.57 min (80–330) for left colectomies and 143.79 min (80–247) for sigmoidectomy. We observed a stabilization of operative times after completion of the team learning curve. In the most recent 50 cases average operative time decreased to 141.3 min and 132.5 min, respectively.

The conversion rate to laparotomy was 1.75% (5/286) as a result of a good standardization of the technique and careful selection of patients for laparoscopy. Conversion to open procedure was more commonly related to disease factors (one Hinchey 4, two severe inflammation, two due to difficulties linked to the exposure of the operative field).

One intraoperative complication (0.34%) was observed: a complete devascularization of the descending colon before completing the colorectal anastomosis. A right colon derotation with middle colic and right colic vessel ligation was performed, followed by a colorectal anastomosis.

Intraoperative blood loss averaged 100 cc (range: 30-180). The average length of operative specimen was 28 cm (range 16-40). Histologic examination revealed three invasive carcinomas (1.04%), two Dukes C and one Dukes A, and one villous adenoma with severe dysplasia (0.34%). No intraoperative mortality was observed and only one death (0.34%) on the 4th postoperative day, due to pulmonary embolism, in spite of routine antithrombotic prophylaxis.

Postoperative complications occurred in 37 patients (12.93%). One had bleeding from the anastomotic staple line (0.34%) which required transanal revision. This patient subsequently developed stenosis of the anastomosis and was successfully treated with endoscopic dilatation. One patient (0.34%) developed peritonitis on the 7th postoperative day due to covered ileal perforation, which required re operation. One patient (0.34%) had postoperative intraperitoneal bleeding which was treated conservatively with a transfusion of 2 units of concentrated red blood cells. Sixteen patients (5.59%) had a suppuration of the mini-laparotomy. Three (1.04%) patients developed an abdominal fluid collection which was drained percutaneously. Seven patients (2.44%) had a urinary tract infection, one (0.34%) a pulmonary infection, one (0.34%) pulmonary embolism.

Six patients (2.09%) developed an anastomotic fistula, which was treated with laparoscopic reoperation, peritoneal lavage, drainage and ileostomy. The average hospital stay was 6.74 days (range 5–22). Patients sent for follow up (mean 48 months) showed no recurrence of diverticulitis, no stricture of anastomosis and no urinary or reproductive system dysfunctions.

6.4 Literature Search Method

The literature search was done using the following criteria:

- Guidelines on the topic published between 1990 and 2010 were taken into consideration, including their references and web pages;
- PubMed was searched with the following criteria:
  - *Limits Activated*: Humans, Clinical Trial, Meta-Analysis, Practice Guideline, Randomized Controlled Trial, Review, English, All Adult: 19+ years, published in the last 5 years
  - *Search details*: [((“laparoscopy”[MeSH Terms] OR “laparoscopic”[All Fields]) AND (“diverticulitis”[MeSH Terms] OR “diverticul*”[All Fields])) AND (“humans”[MeSH Terms] AND (Clinical Trial[ptyp] OR Meta-Analysis[ptyp] OR Practice Guideline[ptyp] OR Randomized

Controlled Trial[ptyp] OR Review[ptyp]) AND English[lang] AND "adult"[MeSH Terms] AND "2005/1/1"[PDat] : "2010/11/25"[PDat])].

A total of 49 abstracts were evaluated, of which 35 were extracted in full-text; papers were selected and classified on the basis of highest evidence design of the study (following Oxford's hierarchy) and most recent publication.

Patients admitted for acute diverticulitis should undergo abdominal CT scan (with i.v. contrast) to further be classified according to Ambrosetti's classification. US may serve as another useful diagnostic tool but has limitations based on experience of examiner and type of patient examined. CT scans have nowadays largely replaced barium enema as the preferred imaging modality to evaluate patients with suspected diverticulitis. (GoR A)

The value of CT scanning for acute diverticulitis is the ability to confirm the diagnosis and to classify the severity of the disease differentiating mild, localized inflammation from severe inflammation with abscess formation and/or diffuse peritonitis [5]. Before the advent of CT, the contrast enema was the primary tool in the evaluation of colonic diverticular disease. However, CT scan has largely replaced barium enema as the preferred imaging technique to evaluate patients with suspected diverticulitis. The use of CT scanning has been justified by several studies, demonstrating a high sensitivity (97%) and specificity (100%) for diverticulitis [5]. Contrast enema, on the other hand, has a sensitivity of only 82% and a specificity of 81% for diverticulitis [10]. The patient, after admission, should therefore be classified for severity and extension of disease using clinical classification, based on symptoms and clinical evaluation [2] and Ambrosetti's classification, based on CT findings [5]. Hinchey's classification and its modifications, on the other hand, provides a classification of severity of disease for clinical description and decision making even though a precise Hinchey classification can only be made intraoperatively (fecal or purulent peritonitis). Hinchey 1 indicates the presence of a pericolic abscess, Hinchey 2a indicates distant abscess amenable to percutaneous drainage, Hinchey 2b indicates complex abscess associated with or without fistula. Diffuse peritonitis is classified as Hinchey 3 (purulent) or 4 (fecal) [2, 11].

If emergency surgery is indicated (Hinchey 3 or 4), the patient's conditions have to be very carefully evaluated to select patients suitable for the laparoscopic approach (fit, stable, non immunocompromised patients with recent peritonitis, no signs of septic shock) and patients to operate directly with a laparotomy (unfit, with multiple comorbidities, unstable, with signs of septic shock), in whom a Hartmann's procedure is preferable.

Elective laparoscopic surgery is an acceptable alternative to conventional surgery for treatment of Hinchey 1, with abscess larger than 5 cm, and in Hinchey 2a patients, after initial conservative treatment with percutaneous drainage of abscess. (GoR A)

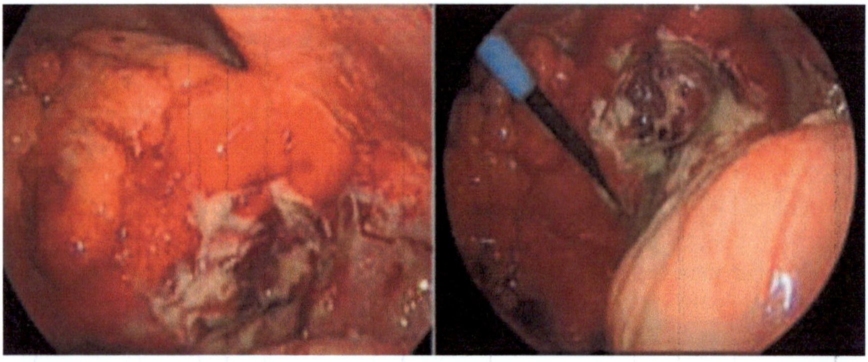

Fig. 6.1 A 48-year-old male patient with peritonitis Hinchey 3. Laparoscopic lavage and drainage after closure of the diverticular defect. Laparoscopic sigmoidectomy three months later. Healing

Laparoscopic surgery is increasingly preferred in the elective treatment of sigmoid diverticulitis. Several single institutional series have confirmed the feasibility and safety of the laparoscopic approach in elective surgery [12–15]. Laparoscopic sigmoidectomy is associated with reduced recovery time, return to bowel function, reduced hospital stay, decreased morbidity [16–18] and costs [18, 19] compared with the open technique. Single institutional series by experienced surgeons have reported conversion rates of 2.8% and a median hospital stay of 4 days [15]. In addition, there is further evidence of the benefits of laparoscopic surgery emerging from a prospective randomized trial, which showed a reduction in major complications after laparoscopic surgery when compared with open sigmoidectomy [6]. Reduction of major complications included intra-abdominal abscess, anastomotic leakage, pulmonary embolism and myocardial infarction.

In the acute setting of disease with peritonitis Hinchey 3 (Fig. 6.1), in patients not amenable to percutaneous drainage of abscesses (Hinchey 2b) or in Hinchey 1 and 2a patients in whom initial conservative management fails, laparoscopic lavage and drainage should be considered in selected cases. (GoR B)

In cases of Hinchey 2b not amenable to percutaneous drainage or Hinchey 3 diverticulitis where either localized or free intra-abdominal pus is present, a limited laparoscopic procedure can be performed with lavage and drainage of the abdominal cavity without bowel resection or formation of a stoma [20]. This aims to convert a generalized purulent peritonitis to a localized diverticulitis which can be safely treated by broad-spectrum antibiotic therapy [21–23]. Once the acute inflammation has settled, a delayed definitive laparoscopic resection in elective setting can be performed, thereby completing the totally minimally invasive management in such patients. In addition to the avoidance of a laparotomy and stoma, this approach allows a definitive colonic resection in a non-emergency situation, which is the current trend [1, 24].

The totally minimally invasive approach seems to be a good alternative strategy for Hinchey 3 that may improve outcomes in a selected group of patients. It does, however, have its limits. There is a risk of early re operation if the initial intervention fails to control the abdominal sepsis because of persistent fistulization despite the closure of the diverticular defect.

It is, therefore, important to have strict criteria for patient selection to obtain good results: patients whose perforation is visible at laparoscopic exploration or Hinchey 4 cases should be excluded from lavage-drainage [7, 21, 25–27]. These patients may benefit from exteriorization of the perforation or from resection with or without a protective stoma [26]. Some authors propose in such cases suturing of the perforation or/and an omental patch or fibrin glue [26] with good results, low complication rate and immediate improvement of clinical conditions [22, 23]. Again, patients whose exploration of the abdomen is not satisfactory because of adhesions or obstruction and when exploration shows severe peritonitis with numerous false membranes or fecal peritonitis should be considered for conversion into open surgery for a standard resection [21, 22, 26] (Hartmann or resection-anastomosis with or without protective stoma).

After peritoneal lavage and drainage, elective sigmoid resection should be planned within 3-6 months. Laparoscopic lavage and drainage has the potential to become in a subgroup of patients the definitive treatment for Hinchey 3. (GoR B)

The initial experiences of laparoscopic lavage and drainage have been promising with respect to perioperative mortality and complication rates [21]. In addition, while most proponents of initial laparoscopic lavage suggest an elective, delayed sigmoidectomy, a multicenter study from Ireland and other small studies reported encouraging results with lavage followed by continued follow-up. In fact, Myers et al. [7] noted recurrence of sigmoid diverticulitis in four out of 92 treated patients, none of whom required surgery after a median follow-up of 36 months. These data coming also from different centers [28, 29] suggest that laparoscopic lavage may become, in selected cases, the definitive treatment for perforated diverticulitis. The explanation could be that an episode of severe diverticulitis may result in a buttressing effect around the affected portion of the colon, thereby protecting it from subsequent attacks [3]. Nevertheless, the number of studies are rather limited and mostly based on small groups of patients, so further investigations are needed to confirm these initial, promising results.

There is still not enough evidence to recommend laparoscopic resection for Hinchey 3-4 patients, even though there is increasing evidence that in selected patients and experienced hands it may be considered potentially safe and effective with no apparent increase in intra- or postoperative complications. (GoR C)

Alternatively to laparoscopic lavage in Hinchey 3–4 patients, emergency colonic resection can be done by laparoscopy in carefully selected cases. The choice between Hartmann and resection-anastomosis with or without protective stoma has to be made on a case-by-case basis [30], based on the patient's conditions and the operator's skills, keeping in mind that Hartmann's procedure should be preferred in unfit patients, with multiple comorbidities, in whom the quality of inflamed tissues does not guarantee a safe anastomosis.

The reported mortality and morbidity in patients with an anastomosis seems to be the same as in patients who undergo the Hartmann procedure [4]. These data suggest that in a select group of patients undergoing surgery in the acute stage of diverticulitis, an anastomosis is probably safe, even in the setting of feculent peritonitis.

When performed laparoscopically, colonic resection in the emergency setting has in some small series [31–34] proven to be effective and safe, although the rates of additional radiologic interventions and conversion to an open procedure are high [27]. Moreover, for many hospitals it will not be possible to have a surgical team with expertise in colorectal laparoscopic surgery present all the time. Therefore, laparoscopy is of unclear or limited value in the emergency setting caused by perforated diverticular disease and there is still not enough evidence to recommend this policy in routine practice.

It is currently considered prudent to exclude from laparoscopic access unfit, unstable patients, with symptoms of septic shock or ASA 3–4 patients, which should be sent directly for a laparotomy.

6.5 Conclusions

After patient admission for diverticulitis an immediate CT scan is of paramount importance to distinguish patients with mild disease from those affected by severe disease (Ambrosetti's classification). This first objective diagnosis of acute diverticulitis is very helpful to better define the indications for emergent or elective surgery or for conservative management with or without percutaneous drainage of abscesses.

If needed, percutaneous drainage of an associated abscess that may allow the surgeon to perform, after the acute disease has settled, an elective single stage resection with a primary bowel anastomosis. If percutaneous drainage fails, laparoscopic lavage and drainage is a good alternative to urgent colonic resection in selected patients, possibly followed by elective laparoscopic resection. The current trend in fact, with the best results in terms of intra- and postoperative complications, is to avoid an operation close to the acute attack, where possible, leaving to emergency surgery only Hinchey 3 and 4 patients and those who fail to respond to conservative management.

Laparoscopic elective resection is currently considered the best choice for the treatment of non acute diverticular disease with evidence level 1b [33, 35, 36].

In the acute setting, a clinical evaluation has to be carefully performed preoperatively in order to select patients for eventual laparoscopic exploration from those to treat directly with a laparotomic approach.

Laparoscopic lavage and drainage has a valid role in the treatment of stable, fit, Hinchey 3 patients in which no gross perforation is visible, with recent peritonitis, providing a time window for definitive elective resection. If these conditions are not respected or if laparoscopic exploration reveals a Hinchey 4, it is considered prudent to convert the patient to laparotomy and to perform a colonic resection. Emergency colonic resection can be done by laparoscopy, in carefully selected cases, as some authors report [31–34], but evidence for a recommendation is actually too weak.

In Hinchey 3 or 4 patients the choice between Hartmann's operation and resection-anastomosis with or without protective stoma has to be made case by case, based on patient conditions and operator skills, keeping in mind that Hartmann's procedure should be limited to unfit, unstable patients, with multiple comorbidities, immunocompromised, or in whom the quality of inflamed tissues does not guarantee a safe anastomosis [37].

Results obtained in our series of 286 patients come from total standardization of the technique by the operating team, which has an overall experience of 1,348 colonic resections at September 2010. Operating times and percentage of conversions decreased as the team's experience grew. Like the current trend in the treatment of complicated diverticular disease, for the most part in our experience surgical treatment is performed electively.

From the technical point of view, a tension-free anastomosis is assured by mobilizing the splenic flexure which is usually done systematically, except in selected cases. The distal dissection is carefully extended to ensure the resection of the diseased colon below the rectosigmoid junction, which is shown to be associated with lower recurrence rates. Laparoscopic colonic resection to remove the diseased segment of the colon but not all diverticula is the recommended procedure.

On the basis of our experience and evidence from the literature it can be stated that surgical treatment of complicated diverticular disease carried out laparoscopically gives good results in terms of morbidity and mortality. Laparoscopy requires its own specific surgical strategy, especially when complicated cases (abscesses, fistula) are operated. The surgical team must be expert in laparoscopic surgery and colorectal surgery and the technique must be standardized so that the incidence of complications, operating time and rates of conversions to open surgery can be minimized.

References

1. Stocchi L (2010) Current indications and role of surgery in the management of sigmoid diverticulitis. World JGastroenterol 16:4-17
2. EAES (1999) EAES Consensus Statement – Diagnosis and treatment of diverticular disease. Surg Endosc 13:430-436

3. Chapman JR, Dozois EJ, Wolff BG et al (2006) Diverticulitis: a progressive disease? Do multiple recurrences predict less favourable outcomes? Ann Surg 243:876-880
4. Salem L, Flum DR (2004) Primary anastomosis or Hartmann's procedure for patients with diverticular peritonitis? A systematic review. Dis Colon Rectum 47:1953-1964
5. Ambrosetti P, Jenny A, Becker C et al (2000) Acute left colonic diverticulitis compared performance of computed tomography and water-soluble contrast enema: prospective evaluation of 420 patients. Dis Colon Rectum 43:1363-1367
6. Klarenbeek BR, Veenhof AA, Bergamaschi R et al (2009) Laparoscopic sigmoid resection for diverticulitis decreases major morbidity rates: a randomized controlled trial: short-term results of the Sigma Trial. Ann Surg 249:39-44
7. Myers E, Kavanagh D, Hurley M et al (2008) Laparoscopic peritoneal lavage for generalized peritonitis due to perforated diverticulitis - A feasible alternative. Dis Colon Rectum 51:13
8. Sartori CA, Balduino M, Dal Pozzo A et al (2003) Laparoscopic colonic resections for diverticular disease. Results of a single center series of 105 patients. Surgical strategy and technique. Osp Ital Chir 9:111-120
9. Sartori CA (2007) Trattato di tecnica chirurgica laparoscopica del colon e del retto. SVP press, Padua
10. Lawrimore T, Rhea J (2004) Computed tomography evaluation of diverticulitis. J Intensive Care Med 19:194-204
11. Hinchey EJ, Schaal PGH, Richards GK (1978) Treatment of perforated diverticular disease of the colon. Adv Surg 12:85-109
12. Pugliese R, Di Lernia S, Sansonna F et al (2004) Laparoscopic treatment of sigmoid diverticulitis: a retrospective review of 103 cases. Surg Endosc 18:1344 1348
13. Schwandner O, Farke S, Fischer F et al (2004) Laparoscopic colectomy for recurrent and complicated diverticulitis: a prospective study of 396 patients. Langenbecks Arch Surg 389:97-103
14. Garrett KA, Champagne BJ, Valerian BT et al (2008) A single training center's experience with 200 consecutive cases of diverticulitis: can all patients be approached laparoscopically? Surg Endosc 22:2503-2508
15. Jones OM, Stevenson AR, Clark D et al (2008) Laparoscopic resection for diverticular disease: follow-up of 500 consecutive patients. Ann Surg 248:1092-1097
16. Faynsod M, Stamos MJ, Arnell T et al (2000) A case-control study of laparoscopic versus open sigmoid colectomy for diverticulitis. Am Surg 66:841-843
17. Dwivedi A, Chahin F, Agrawal S et al (2002) Laparoscopic colectomy vs. open colectomy for sigmoid diverticular disease. Dis Colon Rectum 45:1309-1315
18. Lawrence DM, Pasquale MD, Wasser TE (2003) Laparoscopic versus open sigmoid colectomy for diverticulitis. Am Surg 69:499-504
19. Senagore AJ, Duepree HJ, Delaney CP et al (2002) Cost structure of laparoscopic and open sigmoid colectomy for diverticular disease: similarities and differences. Dis Colon Rectum 45:485-490
20. Mutch MG (2010) Complicated diverticulitis: are there indications for laparoscopic lavage and drainage? Dis Colon Rectum 53:1465-1466
21. O'Sullivan GC, Murphy D, O'Brien MG, Ireland A (1996) Laparoscopic management of generalized peritonitis due to perforated colonic diverticula. Am J Surg 171:432-434
22. Franklin ME Jr, Dorman JP, Jacobs M, Plasencia G (1997) Is laparoscopic surgery applicable to complicated colonic diverticular disease? Surg Endosc 11:1021-1025
23. Da Rold AR, Guerriero S, Fiamingo P et al (2004) Laparoscopic colorrhaphy, irrigation and drainage in the treatment of complicated acute diverticulitis: initial experience. Chir Ital 56:95-98
24. Toorenvliet BR, Swank H, Schoones JW et al (2010) Laparoscopic peritoneal lavage for perforated colonic diverticulitis: a systematic review. Colorectal Dis 12:862-867
25. Bretagnol F, Pautrat K, Mor C et al (2008) Emergency laparoscopic management of perforated sigmoid diverticulitis: a promising alternative to more radical procedures. J Am Coll Surg 206:654-657

26. Faranda C, Barrat C, Catheline JM, Champault GG (2000) Two stage laparoscopic management of generalized peritonitis due to perforated sigmoid diverticula: eighteen cases. Surg Laparosc Endosc Percutan Tech 10:135-141
27. Taylor CJ, Layani L, Ghusn MA, White SI (2006) Perforated diverticulitis managed by laparoscopic lavage. ANZ J Surg 76:962-965
28. Karoui M, Champault A, Pautrat K (2009) Laparoscopic peritoneal lavage or primary anastomosis with defunctioning stoma for Hinchey 3 complicated diverticulitis: results of a comparative study. Dis Colon Rectum 52:609-615
29. Favuzza J, Friel J, Kelly JJ et al (2009) Benefits of laparoscopic peritoneal lavage for complicated sigmoid diverticulitis Int J Colorectal Dis 24:797-801
30. Rafferty J, Shellito P, Hyman NH, Buie WD (2006) Practice parameters for sigmoid diverticulitis. Dis Colon Rectum 49:939-944
31. Agaba EA, Zaidi RM, Ramzy P et al (2009) Laparoscopic Hartmann's procedure: a viable option for treatment of acutely perforated diverticulitis. Surg.Endosc 23:1483-1486
32. Martel G, Bouchard A, Soto CM et al (2010) Laparoscopic colectomy for complex diverticular disease: a justifiable choice? Surg Endosc 24:2273-2280
33. Scheidbach H, Schneider C, Rose J et al (2004) Laparoscopic approach to treatment of sigmoid diverticulitis: changes in the spectrum of indications and results of a prospective, multicenter study on 1,545 patients. Dis Colon Rectum 47:1883-1888
34. Zdichavsky M, Granderath FA, Blumenstock G et al (2010) Acute laparoscopic intervention for diverticular disease: a feasible approach. Langenbecks Arch Surg 395:41-48
35. Gervaz P, Inan I, Perneger T et al (2010) A prospective, randomized, single-blind comparison of laparoscopic versus open sigmoid colectomy for diverticulitis. Ann Surg 252:3-8
36. Pavlidis TE, Pavlidis ET, Sakantamis AK (2010) Current management of diverticular disease of the colon. Tech Coloproctol 14:79-81
37. Tonelli F, Di Carlo V, Liscia G, Serventi A (2009) La malattia diverticolare del colon: quando e come trattarla. Consensus Conference 5° Congresso Nazionale della Società Italiana dei Chirurghi Universitari (SICU). Ann Ital Chir 80:3-8

Suggested Readings

Sauerland S, Agresta F, Bergamaschi R, Borzellino G, Budzynski A, Champault G, Fingerhut A, Isla A, Johansson M, Lundorff P (2006) Laparoscopy for abdominal emergencies. Evidence-based guidelines of the European Association for Endoscopic Surgery. Surg Endosc 20:14–29

Agresta F, Ansaloni L, Baiocchi L, Bergamini C, Campanile FB, Carlucci M, Cocorullo G, Corradi A, Franzato B, Lupo M, Mandalà V, Mirabella A, Pernazza G, Piccoli M, Staudacher C, Vettoretto N, Zago M, Lettieri E, Levati A, Pietrini D, Scaglione M, De Masi S, De Placido G, Francucci M, Rasi M, Scaramuzza G, Del Favero ALl (2011) Consensus Development Conference of the Società Italiana Chirurgia Endoscopica e nuove tecnologie (SICE); Associazione Chirurghi Ospedalieri Italiani (ACOI); Società Italiana di Chirurgia (SIC); Società Italiana Chirurgia d'Urgenza e Trauma (SICUT), Società Italiana Chirurghi dell'Ospedalità Privata (SICOP) and the European Association for Endoscopic Surgery (EAES). In press

Adhesive Small Bowel Obstruction

7

Fausto Catena, Salomone Di Saverio, Luca Ansaloni,
Antonio Pinna, Massimo Lupo, Antonino Mirabella and Vincenzo Mandalà

7.1 Introduction

In recent years, progress in technology and surgical techniques has led to a rapid development in laparoscopic surgery, which is beginning to be frequently used even for several kinds of abdominal emergencies, such as inflammatory syndromes, and more rarely in cases of trauma and bowel obstruction. In the latter, however, the indication for the laparoscopic approach today is debated among surgeons due to the potential visceral risk associated with this method and also because the scientific evidence currently available in the literature supporting the use of the laparoscopic approach over open surgery is poor.

The most recent guidelines for the management of adhesive small bowel obstruction (ASBO) have given the following recommendations for the surgical treatment of ASBO [1]:

- after 3 days of nonoperative treatment without resolution of ASBO surgery is recommended (EL 2c GoR C);
- if ileus persists for more than 3 days and the drainage volume on day 3 is >500 mL, surgery for ASBO is recommended (EL 2b GoR C);
- when fever and leukocytosis level (> 15,000/mm^3) rises anytime during the course, then surgery is advised (GoR C);
- open surgery is the preferred method for the surgical treatment of strangulating ASBO and after failed conservative management (EL 2c GoR C);
- in a highly selected group of patients the laparoscopic approach can be attempted using an open access technique (EL 2c GoR C);
- access in the left upper quadrant should be safe (EL 4 GoR C);

F. Catena (✉)
Department of General Emergency and Transplant Surgery,
"S. Orsola-Malpighi" University Hospital,
Bologna, Italy

V. Mandalà, *The Role of Laparoscopy in Emergency Abdominal Surgery*,

- laparoscopic lysis of adhesions should be attempted preferably in cases of first episode SBO and/or anticipated single band adhesion (i.e. SBO after appendectomy or hysterectomy) (EL 3b GoR C);
- a low threshold for open conversion should be maintained if extensive adhesions are found (EL 2c GoR C);
- conversion to laparoscopic-assisted adhesiolysis (mini-laparotomy with an incision less than 4 cm long) or laparotomy should be considered in those patients presenting with dense or pelvic adhesion (EL 3b GoR C).

7.2 Literature Review

The extent of adhesiolysis is a matter still under debate. The approaches to adhesiolysis for bowel obstruction among general surgeons in the United Kingdom were established in 1993 [2]. Half of all surgeons divided all adhesions to prevent recurrence of bowel obstruction, whereas the other half limited adhesiolysis to only the adhesions responsible for the obstruction.

Adhesions are less after transverse or Pfannenstiel incision than after midline incisions and surgery for obstetric rather than gynecologic indications [3]. The risk of anterior abdominal wall adhesions increases with the number of previous laparotomies, although this relationship is not as evident as the relationship between previous laparotomies and adhesiolysis-induced enterotomy [4, 5].

In a prospective study of 1,791 patients undergoing benign colorectal surgery (n=1,701) or surgery for small bowel obstruction (n=90) with 89% having baseline adhesions, the mean time to lyse adhesions was 34 min (range 1–240 min) [6]. Mean time required for lysis of adhesions was about one-fifth of the total mean operative time. Notably, 34% of patients had no previous abdominopelvic surgery and presented nonsurgical adhesions resulting from intra-abdominal inflammatory and infectious processes associated with benign colorectal diseases including diverticulitis, Crohn's disease and ulcerative colitis.

Higher age and higher number of previous laparotomies appeared to be predictors of the occurrence of inadvertent enterotomy [5]. Patients with three or more previous laparotomies had a 10-fold increase in enterotomy compared with patients with one or two previous laparotomies, which strongly suggests more dense adhesion reformation after each reoperation.

Historically, laparotomy and open adhesiolysis have been the treatment for patients requiring surgery for small bowel obstruction. Unfortunately, this often leads to further formation of intra-abdominal adhesions with approximately 10% to 30% of patients requiring another laparotomy for recurrent bowel obstruction [7].

In animal models laparoscopy has been shown to decrease the incidence, extent, and severity of intra-abdominal adhesions when compared with open surgery, thus potentially decreasing the recurrence rate for adhesive small bowel obstruction [8].

Laparoscopy seems to have an advantage above laparotomy in terms of adhesion formation to the abdominal wall and to the operative site [9, 10].

Laparoscopic adhesiolysis for small bowel obstruction has a number of potential advantages: (1) less postoperative pain; (2) quicker return of intestinal function; (3) shorter hospital stay; (4) reduced recovery time, allowing an earlier return to full activity; (5) fewer wound complications; and (6) decreased postoperative adhesion formation [11].

However, no randomized controlled trial comparing open to laparoscopic adhesiolysis exists to date, and both the precise indications and specific outcomes of laparoscopic adhesiolysis for ASBO remain poorly understood. The only RCT on laparoscopic adhesiolysis assessed the incidence of chronic abdominal pain after randomization to laparoscopic adhesiolysis or no treatment during diagnostic laparoscopy and it failed to demonstrate any significant differences in terms of pain or discomfort [12].

Although data from retrospective clinical controlled trials suggest that laparoscopy seems feasible and better in terms of hospital stay and mortality reduction, high quality randomized controlled trials assessing all clinically relevant outcomes including overall mortality, morbidity, hospital stay and conversion are lacking [13].

Although the adhesiolysis hospitalization rate has remained constant in the USA since 1988, inpatient expenditures have decreased by nearly 10% because of a 15% decrease in the average length of stay (from 11.2 days in 1988 to 9.7 days in 1994) [14]. This large population survey of hospital discharge reports suggests that the less invasive laparoscopic surgical techniques for adhesiolysis have increased over recent years, contributing to the decreased time required in the hospital for both the surgical procedure itself and the recovery time. However, the increased use of laparoscopy during this study period did not appear to be associated with a concomitant reduction in the adhesiolysis hospitalization rate, therefore a common denominator may exist between surgical trauma and immune response to foreign bodies.

When deciding between an open or laparoscopic approach, the first consideration is that the surgeon be trained and capable of performing advanced laparoscopy. With regards to patient selection, patients with an acute small bowel obstruction and peritonitis or free air requiring an emergent operation are best managed with a laparotomy. Patients without peritonitis who do not resolve with nonoperative management should be considered for laparoscopic adhesiolysis. In these cases, it is important to consider the bowel diameter, degree of abdominal distention, and location of the obstruction (i.e. proximal or distal). Suter et al. [15] found that a bowel diameter exceeding 4 cm was associated with an increased rate of conversion: 55% versus 32% (p=0.02). Patients with a distal and complete small bowel obstruction have an increased incidence of intraoperative complications and increased risk of conversion. Patients with persistent abdominal distention after nasogastric intubation are also unlikely to be treated successfully with laparoscopy.

The influence of dense adhesions and number of previous operations on the success of laparoscopic adhesiolysis is controversial. León et al. [16] state that a documented history of severe or extensive dense adhesions is a contraindication to laparoscopy. Navez et al. [17] found that patients who had only a previous appendectomy were most likely to be successfully managed with laparoscopy. In contrast, Suter et al. [15] found no correlation between the number and or type of previous surgeries and the chance of a successful laparoscopic surgery. Other factors such as an elevated white blood cell count or fever have not been demonstrated to correlate with an increased conversion rate [15, 17]. One group of patients who are good candidates for laparoscopic adhesiolysis are those with a non-resolving, partial small bowel obstruction or a recurrent, chronic small bowel obstruction demonstrated on contrast study [16, 18].

A recent series of 46 patients [19], showed that the best results in terms of success rate (91.3%) and no intraoperative bowel perforations, with a recurrence-free rate of 93.5% after a mean follow up of 46.5 months, can be achieved in ceratin conditions. These include laparoscopic approach when it is used for subgroups of patients with recurrent SBO after abdominal or pelvic surgery, who arescheduled for elective adhesiolysis or if the laparoscopic intervention is performed early when the patient has failed to respond to 24 h of conservative treatment from the onset of acute SBO.

Perforated or gangrenous bowel is best managed with conversion to either a minilaparotomy or a formal laparotomy. Matted small bowel loops and dense adhesions are also best managed with a formal laparotomy. Navez et al. [17] reported that only 10% of obstructions caused by dense adhesions could be treated successfully with laparoscopy. On the other hand, when the cause of obstruction was a single band, laparoscopic adhesiolysis was successful 100% of the time [17] (Fig. 7.1a, b).

When other etiologies are found, such as internal hernia, inguinal hernia, neoplasm, inflammatory bowel disease, intussusception and gallstone ileus, conversion to a minilaparotomy or a formal laparotomy is required.

Inadvertent enterotomy during reopening of the abdomen or subsequent adhesion dissection is a feared complication of surgery after previous laparotomy. The incidence can be as high as 20% in open surgery and between 1% and 100% in laparoscopy [20].

The incidence of intraoperative enterotomies during laparoscopic adhesiolysis ranges from 3% to 17.6%, with most authors reporting an incidence of about 10% [21, 22]. Suter et al. [15] reported an intraoperative enterotomy incidence of 15.6%, of which 62% were repaired laparoscopically. One of the most dreaded complications of surgery is a missed enterotomy. Although a missed enterotomy can occur after laparotomy, the incidence is higher after laparoscopic surgery. Again Suter et al. [15] reported 4 of 47 cases (8.5%) of missed enterotomies requiring reoperation. In the review of Ghosheh and Salameh [23], the rate of small bowel perforation in laparoscopic surgery for SBO was 6.5%. In the study by Dindo et al. [24] the rate of 4.7% was comparable, although only 1.3% of the perforations were missed intraoperatively. This demonstrates the feasibility and effectiveness of the laparoscopic approach in selected cases of ASBO.

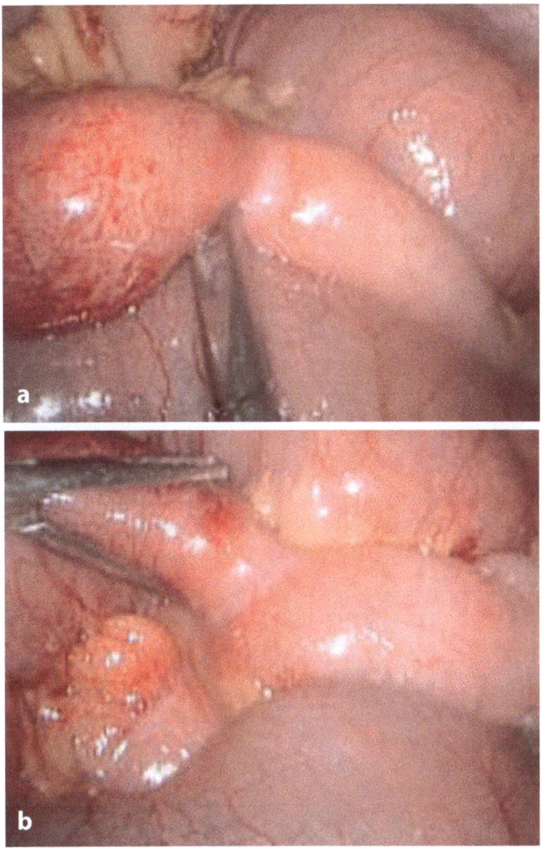

Fig. 7.1a, b Clear view of the transition point at the level of the pinched area. The mark of strangulation on the bowel wall and on the mesentery is visible as well as the distended ischemic proximal loop and the normal distal loop which begins to fill. Courtesy of Salomone Di Saverio MD

The long-term results regarding recurrence are limited, with most series reporting a mean follow-up between 12 and 24 months. Navez et al. [17] reported that 85% (29 of 34) of the patients treated laparoscopically were asymptomatic with a mean follow-up of 46 months. The series with the longest follow-up (mean 61.7 months) reported that 87.5% (14 of 16) of the patients treated laparoscopically were asymptomatic [23].

The feasibility of diagnostic laparoscopy ranges from 60% to 100% whilst therapeutic effectiveness of the laparoscopic approach is lower (40-88%). Predictive factors for successful laparoscopic adhesiolysis are: number of previous laparotomies ≤2; non-median previous laparotomy; appendectomy as previous surgical treatment causing adherences; single band adhesion as pathogenetic mechanism of small bowel obstruction; early laparoscopic management within 24 h from the onset of symptoms; no signs of peritonitis on physical examination; and experience of the surgeon [24].

Surgical operating time is greater in patients who undergo laparoscopic surgery compared to patients who undergo a laparotomy [25, 26]. However, the duration of the laparoscopic procedure is variable, ranging from 20 minutes for a simple band adhesion to 2–3 hours for more complex cases [27, 28]. Postoperative morbidity is lower in patients who undergo laparoscopic adhesiolysis compared to those who undergo the laparotomic approach. Furthermore, a greater rate of morbidity is present in patients who undergo laparotomic conversion, whereas mortality is comparable in the two groups (0–4%). Lastly, laparoscopic adhesiolysis can avoid laparotomy, which is itself a cause of new adhesions and bowel obstruction, although some authors have noticed a greater incidence of recurrent small bowel obstructions in patients who undergo laparoscopy compared to those in which a laparotomy is performed [28–31].

In a large review of 308 patients from 35 centers [32] over 8 years the *successful* laparoscopy rate was 54.6% and the conversion to laparotomy rate was 45.4%. There were significantly more successes among patients with a history of one or two laparotomies than among those with three or more (56% vs. 37%; $p<0.05$). Furthermore, the rate of success was significantly higher ($p<0.001$) in patients operated on early (<24 h) and in patients with bands (54%) than in those with matted adhesions (31%).

In a French experience the laparoscopic approach, with a conversion rate of 31%, did not show any influence on the early postoperative mortality ($p=0.7$) nor on morbidity ($p=0.4$) [32].

Although a laparoscopic approach has been proposed to decrease incisional trauma and to lower the rate of recurrence, a slightly higher but nonstatistically significant rate of recurrences in the laparoscopic approach has been observed. Probably, several additional even smaller incisions and a mandatory identical parietal and visceral adhesiolysis as with laparotomy do not decrease the magnitude of the peritoneal trauma [33].

The largest and most significant population review from the US identified from the 2002 National Inpatient Sample 6,165 patients with intestinal obstruction undergoing open (OLA) and laparoscopic lysis of adhesions (LLA) [34]. Of these 88.6% underwent OLA and 11.4% had LLA. Conversion was required in 17.2% of LLA patients. Unadjusted mortality was equal between LLA and conversion (1.7%) and half the rate compared with OLA (3.4%) ($p=0.014$). The odds of complications in the LLA group (intention to treat) were 25% less than in the OLA ($p=0.008$). The LLA group had a 27% shorter length of surgery ($p=0.0001$) and was 9% less expensive than the OLA group ($p=0.0003$). There was no statistical significant difference for length of surgery, complications, and costs between the conversion and OLA groups.

The comparably low conversion rate of 17% by Mancini et al. [34] in this study may be explained by the low initial percentage (11%) of patients treated laparoscopically, indicating a positive selection of patients amenable to successful laparoscopic adhesiolysis.

Szomstein et al. [35] summarized data on conversion rates for laparoscopic lysis of adhesions and reported a range from 6.7% to 41%. The benefits and advantages of the laparoscopic approach for lysis of adhesions are highlighted in this review of 11 series including 813 patients. They found that 63% of the length of a laparotomy incision is involved in adhesion formation to the abdominal wall. Furthermore, the incidence of ventral hernia after a laparotomy ranges between 11% and 20% versus the 0.02%–2.4% incidence of port site herniation. Additional benefits of the minimally invasive approach include a decreased incidence of wound infection and postoperative pneumonia and a more rapid return of bowel function resulting in a shorter hospital stay. In long-term follow up, the success rate of laparoscopic lysis of adhesions remains between 46% and 87%. Operative times for laparoscopy range from 58 to 108 minutes; conversion rates range from 6.7% to 43%; and the incidence of intraoperative enterotomy ranges from 3% to 17.6%. The length of hospitalization is 4–6 days in most series. In this review again contraindications to the minimally invasive technique include the following: (1) massive abdominal distension that precludes entry into the peritoneal space and limits adequate working space; (2) the presence of peritonitis with the need for bowel resection and bowel handling in a highly inflamed environment; (3) hemodynamic instability; (4) severe comorbid conditions such as heart and lung diseases that preclude the use of pneumoperitoneum; and (5) lastly, but certainly not the least important, the surgeon's comfort level.

An interesting although small review of 93 patients with ASBO from a community teaching hospital [36], divided into successful laparoscopy (66 patients, 71%), secondary conversion (24 patients, 26%), and primary laparotomy (three patients), showed that patients with successful laparoscopy had more simple adhesions (57%), fewer prior operations, and lower ASA class. Operative time was shortest in the laparoscopy group (74.3±4.4 min), as was the duration of both intensive care unit and hospital stay. Mortality was 6%, regardless of operative technique. The author's conclusion confirmed that the parameters associated with successful laparoscopic management of SBO are the presence of isolated bands, lower ASA scores, younger age, fewer prior operations, and a shorter duration of SBO obstruction before the operation. Reasons for primary laparotomy included a state of prolonged ileus with progressive abdominal distension and a higher number or more extensive previous operations. Reasons for converting to open adhesiolysis following initial laparoscopy were inadequate laparoscopic control due to intestinal distension, extensive adhesions, iatrogenic intestinal perforation and the presence of necrotic segments of the small bowel upon initial laparoscopy, requiring secondary open resection.

Zerey et al. [37] reported a series of 33 patients who underwent laparoscopic adhesiolysis secondary to SBO. Twenty-nine patients (88%) were successfully treated laparoscopically. Mean procedural time was 101 minutes (range, 19–198 minutes). Only one patient had a recurrent SBO 8 months postoperatively which was managed by repeat laparoscopic lysis of adhesions. Mean postoperative stay was 6 days.

In another report of 65 patients submitted to laparoscopic adhesiolysis (40 for acute obstruction and 25 for chronic or recurrent transit disturbances), the procedure was completed by laparoscopy in 52 patients (conversion rate: 20%) and after a mean follow up of 48 months a 15.4% rate of symptomatic recur-

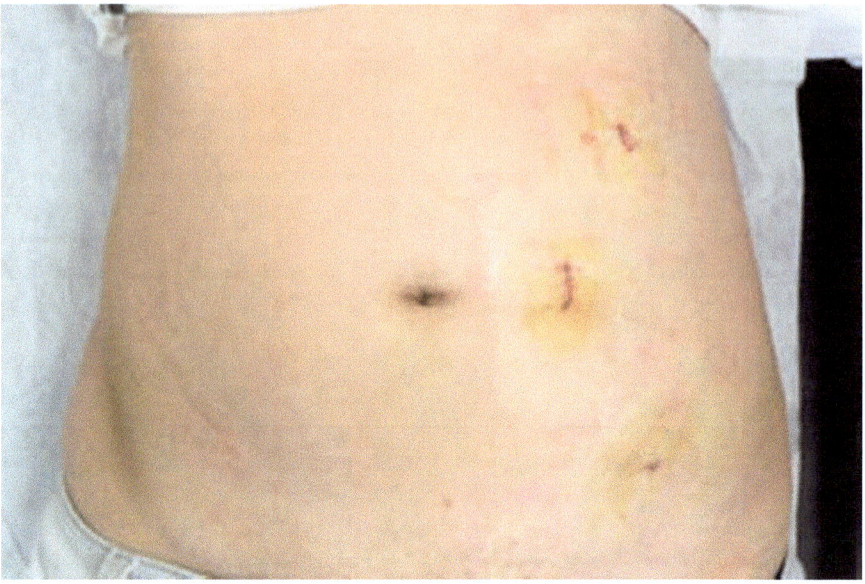

Fig. 7.2 View of the 3-port accesses in the left flank and the visible scar of the previous appendectomy at McBurney's point. Courtesy of Salomone Di Saverio, MD

rences was observed, while surgical recurrences were 4.6% [38].

In a series of 17 patients scheduled for elective adhesiolysis [21], laparoscopic treatment was successful in 14 patients (82.4%) and two recurrences of small bowel obstructions were noted over a mean follow-up period of 61.7 months. In a similar series of elective laparoscopic treatment of 25 patients with recurrent small bowel obstruction, complete laparoscopic adhesiolysis was feasible in 18 patients (72%) and no recurrence of small bowel obstruction over a mean follow-up period of 41 months was observed [39]. In this series conversion to laparoscopic-assisted adhesiolysis (mini-laparotomy with an incision less than 4 cm long) was required in 6 patients (24%) because of dense adhesion or the technical difficulties due to adhesion in the pelvic cavity.

Leon et al. [16] reported a 35% conversion rate in a series of 40 patients and at median follow-up of 12 months, 21 of 26 patients managed laparoscopically or with laparoscopic-assisted procedures remained asymptomatic [16].

A review in 2007 showed that laparoscopic management of SBO is successful in 66% of patients with a conversion rate of 33.5% [37].

Operative technique plays a paramount role in successful laparoscopic treatment [11]. The initial trocar should be placed away (alternative site technique) from the scars in an attempt to avoid adhesions (Fig. 7.2). Some investigators have recommended the use of computed tomography scan or ultrasonography to help determine a safe site for the initial trocar insertion.

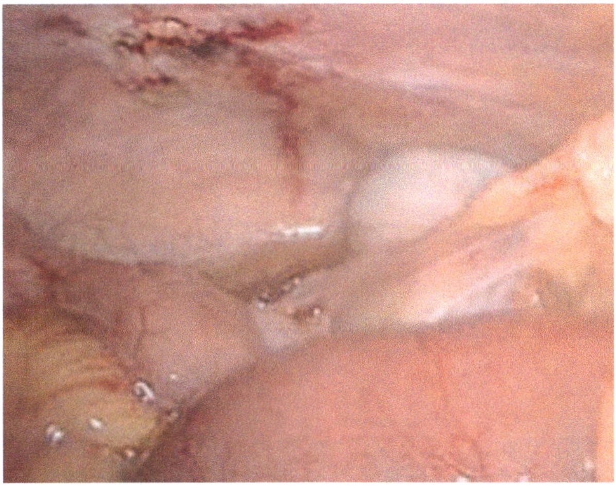

Fig. 7.3 Diagnostic laparoscopy: considerable amount of abdominal free fluid is found. The bowel exploration begins by identifying the cecum and running the collapsed bowel proximally. Courtesy of Salomone Di Saverio, MD

The left upper quadrant is often a safe place to gain access to the abdominal cavity. Alternatively a 10 mm port can be inserted in the left flank with two additional 5 mm ports in the left upper and lower quadrant (Fig. 7.2). Therefore, by triangulating 3 ports aimed at the right lower quadrant, a good exposure and access to the right iliac fossa can be obtained with a technique running the small bowel in a retrograde fashion, starting from the ileocecal valve (decompressed intestine) proximally towards the transition point between collapsed and dilated loops (Fig. 7.3).

The open (Hasson) approach under direct vision is the more prudent. Once safe access is obtained, the next goal is to provide adequate visualization in order to insert the remaining trocars. This often requires some degree of adhesiolysis along the anterior abdominal wall. Numerous techniques are available, including finger dissection through the initial trocar site and using the camera to bluntly dissect the adhesions. Sometimes, gentle retraction on the adhesions will separate the tissue planes (Fig. 7.4a). Most often sharp adhesiolysis is required (Fig. 7.4b). The use of cautery and ultrasound dissection should be limited in order to avoid thermal tissue damage and bowel injury.

Strickland et al. [40] have reported an incidence of 10% enterotomies during exploration and adhesiolysis in 40 patients treated laparoscopically for acute SBO. However an even higher proportion of the patients had enterotomies after conversion (23%) [40]. Furthermore, formal laparotomy was avoided in 68% of these patients and earlier return of bowel function and a shorter postoperative length of stay, with lower overall costs was achieved with laparoscopic treatment. The risk of enterotomy can be reduced if meticulous care is taken in the use of atraumatic graspers only and if the manipulation of friable, distended bowel is minimized by handling the mesentery of the bowel whenever possible (Fig. 7.5). In fact, handling dilated and edematous bowel during adhesiol-

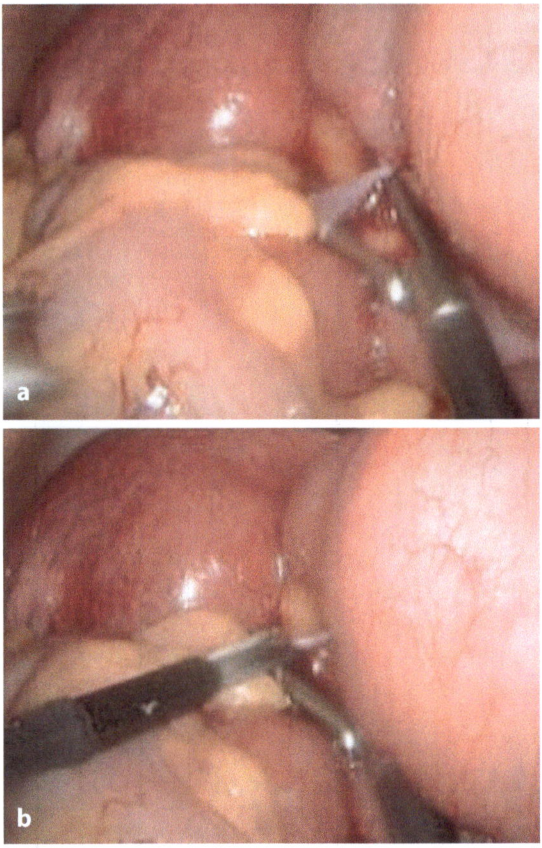

Fig. 7.4a, b Identification of the pelvic single fibrous band adhesion in the right iliac fossa. Sharp dissection with scissors after appropriate lifting up of the band and carefully avoiding use of coagulation. Courtesy of Salomone Di Saverio, MD

ysis is dangerous and the risk increases with a long lasting obstruction; therefore early operation is advisable, with one multicenter study showing that the success rate for early laparoscopic intervention for acute SBO was significantly higher after a shorter duration of symptoms (24 h vs. 48 h) [31].

Maintaining a low threshold for conversion to laparotomy in the face of extensive adhesions will further decrease the risk of bowel injury.

After trocar placement, the initial goal is to expose the collapsed distal bowel. This is facilitated with the use of angled telescopes and maximal tilting/rotating of the surgical table. It may also be necessary to move the laparoscope to different trocars to improve visualization. If necessary, the small bowel mesentery (instead of the bowel wall) should be grasped in order to manipulate the bowel (Fig. 7.5). Sharp dissection with the laparoscopic scissors should be used to cut the adhesions (Fig. 7.4b). Only pathologic adhesions should be lysed. Additional adhesiolysis only adds to the operative time and to the risks of surgery without benefit. The area lysed should be thoroughly inspected for possible bleeding and bowel injury (Fig. 7.1a, b).

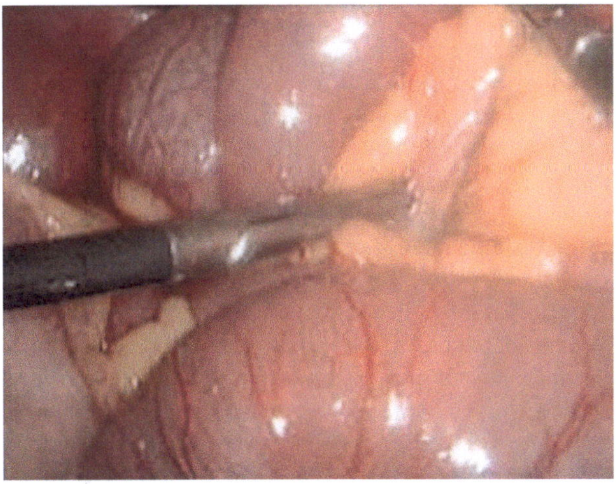

Fig. 7.5 Diagnostic laparoscopy: grasping the distended bowel must be avoided and the mesentery should be gently grasped. Courtesy of Salomone Di Saverio, MD

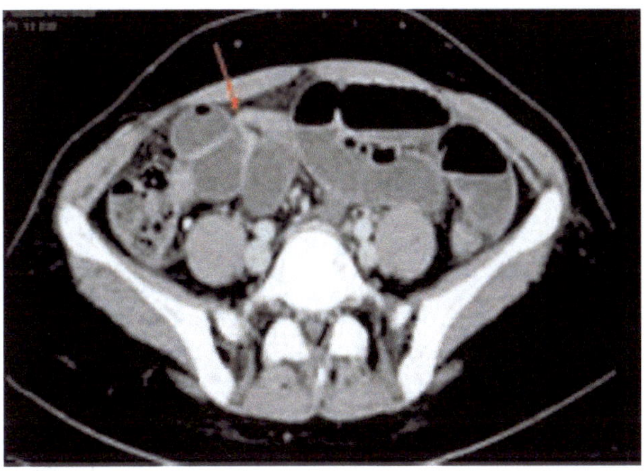

Fig. 7.6 CT finding of complete SBO with a clear transition point in the right iliac fossa and suspected single band (*red arrow*) in a 36-year old patient with history of previous open appendectomy. Courtesy of Salomone Di Saverio, MD

In conclusion, careful selection criteria for laparoscopy [41] may be: (1) proximal obstruction, (2) partial obstruction, (3) anticipated single band, (4) localized distension on radiography, (5) no sepsis, (6) mild abdominal distension and last but not least (7) the experience and laparoscopic skills of the surgeon.

The experts panel also agreed, as from the cited studies, that laparoscopic lysis of adhesions should be attempted preferably in cases of first episode SBO and/or anticipated single band adhesion (i.e. SBO after appendectomy or hysterectomy) (Fig. 7.6).

Furthermore, the experts highlighted that an open port access should be attempted, and gaining the access in the left upper quadrant should be safe.

However, a large consensus has been reached in recommending a low threshold for open conversion if extensive adhesions are found.

Conversion is not a sign of failure; instead, it represents good clinical judgment. Conversion has not been shown to correlate with the number of previous surgeries [17]. However, it may be predicted by bowel distension over 4 cm, a documented history of dense adhesions, and the presence of complete distal obstruction [11]. The main causes for laparotomic conversion are: kind of adhesions, bowel necrosis and accidental enterotomies. In the literature: *if the surgeon notices ischemic or necrotic bowel he must perform a laparotomy.*

In order to reduce the number of conversions some surgeons perform a hand-assisted laparoscopy in selected cases since laparoscopy can also allow a guided laparotomic approach in case of conversion (tailored mini-laparotomy) and a hand-assisted approach, in our experience, can allow the removal of adhesions with a blunt technique especially posterior peritoneal band adhesions impossible to manage with pure laparoscopy [39] (Tsumura's classification).

7.3 Personal Experience

Between February 1999 and February 2011 a total of 178 patients were admitted to the Surgical Centre of Villa Sofia Hospital in Palermo and operated on in emergencies or in deferred emergencies. Of these, 100 (56.1%) had conventional surgical management (by laparotomy) and 78 (43.9%) by laparoscopic approach.

The series included 61 females (61%) (mean age 65.06 years) and 39 males (39%) (mean age 68.27 years) who were treated with conventional surgery and 49 females (62.8%) (mean age 46.79) and 29 males (37.2%) who were treated with the laparoscopic approach. The ages ranged from 27 to 98 years for open procedure and from 23 to 72 years for laparoscopy (Tables 7.1-7.2).

In accordance with the literature most of the cases performed with the laparoscopic approach were secondary to previous appendectomies (27 cases – 34.6%), followed by gynecologic operations (18 cases – 23.1%), two patients had adhesiolysis after open cholecystectomy, in one case after iatrogenic colonic perforation, one case after left nephrectomy and appendectomy, one case the result of subtotal gastrectomy for ulcer, five after a treatment for strangulated femoral hernias, eight after a previous ileocolic resection for Crohn's disease and colonic cancer in nine cases for treatment of unrecognized eventration, four for incisional hernia, one for ileal GIST and one for Meckel's diverticulum.

The conversion rate was 14.1% (11 cases), with one case for iatrogenic injury and one case to check bowel loop integrity; in nine cases (11.5%) we performed a *tailored laparotomy*. In five cases (6.41%) a *hand-assisted* technique was performed (Table 7.3).

The total rate of conversion was therefore 25.6% (32% hand assisted) dis-

Table 7.1 Ileal obstruction, 100 cases which had conventional surgical management (by laparotomy). Department of Emergency Surgery, Villa Sofia Hospital, Palermo

Sex	N	Mean age	%	Hospital stay
Female	61	65.06	54.34	6.25 days
Male	39	68.27	45.66	
		Age range: 27-98		
		Postoperative stay range: 3-24 days		

Table 7.2 Ileal obstruction, 78 cases treated with laparoscopic approach. Department of Emergency Surgery, Villa Sofia Hospital, Palermo

Sex	N	Mean age	%	Hospital stay
Female	49	46.79	60.0	2.38 days
Male	29	42.53	40.0	
		Age range: 23-72		
		Postoperative stay range: 1-8 days		

Table 7.3 Laparoscopic treatment, conversion rates. Department of Emergency Surgery, Villa Sofia Hospital, Palermo

Treatment	N	%
Open surgery	11	14.1
Tailored laparotomy	9	11.5
Hand-assisted technique	5	6.4
Total	25	32

tributed as follows: six cases of dense adhesions; four cases of inadequate visualization; one case of iatrogenic injury; six cases requiring bowel resection; two cases of hernia (one to check bowel loop integrity); one case of unidentified etiology.

The morbidity in cases performed by the laparoscopic approach was eight cases (10.2%) against 19 cases (19%) performed by conventional surgery (Table 7.4). Hospital stay was 2.38 days (1–8 days) in patients treated by laparoscopy, whereas it was 6.25 days (3–24 days) in patients operated on by laparotomy.

Table 7.4 Morbidity: laparoscopic approach vs. open surgery. Department of Emergency Surgery, Villa Sofia Hospital, Palermo

Treatment	N	%
Laparoscopy	8	10.2
Open surgery	19	24.3

References

1. Catena F, Di Saverio S, Kelly MD et al (2011) Bologna Guidelines for Diagnosis and Management of Adhesive Small Bowel Obstruction (ASBO): 2010 Evidence-Based Guidelines of the World Society of Emergency Surgery. World J Emerg Surg 6:5
2. Scott-Coombes DM, Vipond MN, Thompson JM (1993) General surgeons attitudes to the treatment and prevention of abdominal adhesions. Ann R Coll Surg Engl 75:123–128
3. Brill AI, Nezhat F, Nezhat CH, Nezhat C (1995) The incidence of adhesion after prior laparotomy: a laparoscopic appraisal. Obstet Gynecol 85:269–272
4. Levrant SG, Bieber E, Barnes R (1994) Risk of anterior abdominal wall adhesions increases with number and type of previous laparotomy. J Am Assoc Gynecol Laparosc 1:S19
5. Van Der Krabben AA, Dijkstra FR, Nieuwenhuijzen M (2000) Morbidity and mortality of inadvertent enterotomy during adhesiolysis. Br J Surg 87:467–471
6. Fazio VW, Cohen Z, Fleshman JW et al (2006) Reduction in adhesive small-bowel obstruction by Seprafilm adhesion barrier after intestinal resection. Dis Colon Rectum 49:1–11
7. J. Landercasper TH, Cogbill WH, Merry WH et al (1993) Long-term outcome after hospitalization for small-bowel obstruction. Arch Surg 128:765–770
8. Tittel A, Treutner KH, Titkova S et al (2001) Comparison of adhesion reformation after laparoscopic and conventional adhesiolysis in an animal model. Langenbeck's Arch Surg 386:141–145
9. Gamal EM, Metzger P, Szabo G et al (2001) The influence of intraoperative complications on adhesion formation during laparoscopic and conventional cholecystectomy in an animal model. Surg Endosc 15:873–877
10. Gadallah MF, Torres-Rivera C, Ramdeen G et al (2001) Relationship between intraperitoneal bleeding, adhesions, and peritoneal dialysis catheter failure: a method of prevention. Adv Perit Dial 17:127–129
11. Nagle A, Ujiki M, Denham W, Murayama K (2004) Laparoscopic adhesiolysis for small bowel obstruction. Am J Surg 187:464–470
12. Swank DJ, Swank-Bordewijk SC, Hop WC et al (2003) Laparoscopic adhesiolysis in patients with chronic abdominal pain: a blinded randomised controlled multi-centre trial. Lancet 361:1247–1251
13. Cirocchi R, Abraha I, Farinella E et al (2010) Laparoscopic versus open surgery in small bowel obstruction. Cochrane Database Syst Rev 2:CD007511. Review
14. Ray NF, Denton WG, Thamer M et al (1998) Abdominal adhesiolysis: inpatient care and expenditures in the United States in 1994. J Am Coll Surg 186:1–9
15. Suter M, Zermatten P, Hakic N et al (2000) Laparoscopic management of mechanical small bowel obstruction: are there predictors of success or failure? Surg Endosc 14:478–484
16. León EL, Metzger A, Tsiotos GG et al (1998) Laparoscopic management of small bowel obstruction: indications and outcomes. J Gastrointest Surg 2:132–140
17. Navez B, Arimont JM, Guit P (1998) Laparoscopic approach in acute small bowel obstruction. A review of 68 patients. Hepatogastroenterology 45:2146–2150
18. Pekmezci S, Altinli E, Saribeyoglu K et al (2001) Enteroclysis-guided laparoscopic adhesiolysis in recurrent adhesive small bowel obstructions. Surg Laparosc Endosc Percutan Tech 12:165–170
19. Wang Q, Hu ZQ, Wang WJ et al (2009) Laparoscopic management of recurrent adhesive small-bowel obstruction: Long-term follow-up. Surg Today 39:493–499
20. Van Goor H (2007) Consequences and complications of peritoneal adhesions. Colorectal Dis 9[Suppl 2]:25–34
21. Sato Y, Ido K, Kumagai M et al (2001) Laparoscopic adhesiolysis for recurrent small bowel obstruction: long-term follow-up. Gastrointest Endosc 54:476–479
22. Chosidow D, Johanet H, Montario T et al (2000) Laparoscopy for acute small-bowel obstruction secondary to adhesions. J Laparoendosc Adv Surg Tech 10:155–159
23. Ghosheh B, Salameh JR (2007) Laparoscopic approach to acute small bowel obstruction: review of 1061 cases. Surg Endosc 21:1945–1949

24. Dindo D, Schafer M, Muller MK et al (2010) Laparoscopy for small bowel obstruction: the reason for conversion matters. Surg Endosc 24:792-797
25. Farinella E, Cirocchi R, La Mura F et al (2009) Feasibility of laparoscopy for small bowel obstruction. World J Emerg Surg 4:3
26. Wullstein C, Gross E (2003) Laparoscopic compared with conventional treatment of acute adhesive small bowel obstruction. Br J Surg 90:1147–1151
27. Khaikin M, Schneidereit N, Cera S et al (2007) Laparoscopic vs. open surgery for acute adhesive small-bowel obstruction: patient outcome and cost-effectiveness. Surg Endosc 21:742–746
28. Franklin ME, Gonzales JJ, Miter DB et al (2004) Laparoscopic diagnosis and treatment of intestinal obstruction. Surg Endosc 18:26–30
29. Franklin ME, Dorman JP, Pharand D (1994) Laparoscopic surgery in acute small obstruction. Surg Laparosc Endosc 4:289–296
30. Peschaud F, Alves A, Berdah S et al (2006) Indicazioni alla laparoscopia in chirurgia generale e digestiva. J Chir 6:65–79
31. Levard H, Boudet MJ, Msika S et al (2001) French Association for Surgical Research: Laparoscopic treatment of acute small bowel obstruction: a multicentre retrospective study. ANZ J Surg 71:641–646
32. Duron JJ, du Montcel ST, Berger A (2008) French Federation for Surgical Research. Prevalence and risk factors of mortality and morbidity after operation for adhesive postoperative small bowel obstruction. Am J Surg 195:726–734
33. Duron JJ, Silva NJ, du Montcel ST et al (2006) Adhesive postoperative small bowel obstruction: incidence and risk factors of recurrence after surgical treatment: a multicenter prospective study. Ann Surg 244:750–757
34. Mancini GJ, Petroski GF, Lin WC et al (2008) Nationwide impact of laparoscopic lysis of adhesions in the management of intestinal obstruction in the US. J Am Coll Surg 207:520–526
35. Szomstein S, Lo Menzo E, Simpfendorfer C et al (2006) Laparoscopic lysis of adhesions. World J Surg 30:535–540
36. Grafen FC, Neuhaus V, Schöb O, Turina M (2010) Management of acute small bowel obstruction from intestinal adhesions: indications for laparoscopic surgery in a community teaching hospital. Langenbecks Arch Surg 395:57–63
37. Zerey M, Sechrist CW, Kercher KW et al (2007) Laparoscopic management of adhesive small bowel obstruction. Am Surg 73:773–778
38. Borzellino G, Tasselli S, Zerman G et al (2004) Laparoscopic approach to postoperative adhesive obstruction. Surg Endosc 18:686–690
39. Tsumura H, Ichikawa T, Murakami Y, Sueda T (2004) Laparoscopic adhesiolysis for recurrent postoperative small bowel obstruction. Hepatogastroenterology 51:1058–1061
40. Strickland P, Lourie DJ, Suddleson EA et al (1999) Is laparoscopy safe and effective for treatment of acute small-bowel obstruction? Surg Endosc 13:695–698
41. Duh QY (1998) Small bowel obstruction. In: Toouli J, Gossot D, Hunter JG (eds) Endosurgery. Churchill Livingstone, New York pp. 425–431

Suggested Readings

Sauerland S, Agresta F, Bergamaschi R, Borzellino G, Budzynski A, Champault G, Fingerhut A, Isla A, Johansson M, Lundorff P (2006) Laparoscopy for abdominal emergencies. Evidence-based guidelines of the European Association for Endoscopic Surgery. Surg Endosc 20:14–29

Agresta F, Ansaloni L, Baiocchi L, Bergamini C, Campanile FB, Carlucci M, Cocorullo G, Corradi A, Franzato B, Lupo M, Mandalà V, Mirabella A, Pernazza G, Piccoli M, Staudacher C, Vettoretto N, Zago M, Lettieri E, Levati A, Pietrini D, Scaglione M, De Masi S, De Placido G, Francucci M, Rasi M, Scaramuzza G, Del Favero AL (2011) Consensus Development Conference of the Società Italiana Chirurgia Endoscopica e nuove tecnologie (SICE); Associazione

Chirurghi Ospedalieri Italiani (ACOI); Società Italiana di Chirurgia (SIC); Società Italiana Chirurgia d'Urgenza e Trauma (SICUT), Società Italiana Chirurghi dell'Ospedalità Privata (SICOP) and the European Association for Endoscopic Surgery (EAES). In press

Catena F, Di Saverio S, Kelly MD, Biffl WL, Ansaloni L, Mandalà V, Velmahos GC, Sartelli M, Tugnoli G, Lupo M, Mandalà S, Pinna AD, Sugarbaker PH, Van Goor H, Moore EE, Jeekel J (2011) Bologna Guidelines for Diagnosis and Management of Adhesive Small Bowel Obstruction (ASBO): 2010 Evidence-Based Guidelines of the World Society of Emergency Surgery. World J Emerg Surg 6:5

Meinero M (2004) Sindromi aderenziali in chirurgia addominale: relazione biennale. Società italiana di chirurgia, Roma

Incarcerated Hernia

8

Micaela Piccoli, Grazia M. Attinà, Domenico Marchi,
Vincenzo Trapani and Gianluigi Melotti

8.1 Introduction

Laparoscopic repair of inguinal, ventral and incisional hernia has gained wider acceptance among surgeons than the open technique, due to the favorable results in terms of incidence of recurrences, complications and patient satisfaction. Most of the series published in the literature concern elective cases. In contrast, the role of laparoscopy in the treatment of incarcerated or strangulated hernias has not been yet established because of the small number of case series. After postoperative peritoneal adhesions, these diseases are the second most common cause of occlusion of the small intestine and therefore deserve separate consideration [1].

8.2 Incarcerated Inguinal Hernia

The probability of an inguinal hernia incarcerating varies considerably, from 0.29% to 2.9% in the literature [2]. The condition can cause intestinal obstruction or strangulation and infarction, resulting in a high incidence of infection, recurrence and operative mortality, especially in the elderly [3].

Elective surgery for inguinal hernia has a very low mortality (<1 death for 10,000 operations). In contrast, the risks of postoperative complications following emergency surgery, especially in elderly patients, are high with a mortality that can be as high as 5% [2].

Elective laparoscopic inguinal hernia repair introduced in the late 1990s by Schultz et al. [4] has been well documented in the literature and it has gradu-

G.M. Attinà (✉)
Department of Surgery, "S. Agostino-Estense" New Hospital
Modena, Italy

ally gained acceptance. It is indicated primarily for bilateral and recurrent hernias and relatively contraindicated for patients with prior operations involving the preperitoneal area such as prostatectomy, large inguinoscrotal hernias or a general condition that prohibits general anesthesia [5].

It was not until 2003 that the first evidence based study by the Cochrane Library appeared, which showed that the laparoscopic technique typically offers less pain and scarring, a more rapid return to work and other activities, a low rate of conversion to open surgery and a short hospital stay [6]. However, operation times are longer and the risk of serious complications with respect to visceral (especially bladder) and vascular injuries is higher [7, 8].

The use of laparoscopy for acute or chronic incarcerated inguinal hernia has been a controversial issue, with some surgeons showing caution in using this technique. Traditionally, incarcerated inguinal hernia has been treated with conventional open techniques. This condition is traditionally considered a contraindication to laparoscopic repair, for several reasons: the increased risk of mesh infection (positioned preperitoneally), the technical difficulties encountered in reducing the hernia sac and its contents and the increased risk of iatrogenic injuries [2, 5].

In 1993 Watson et al. [9] published the first case report of an inguinal hernia laparoscopic reduction combined with a bowel resection. After that, several authors explored the feasibility of using this approach for incarcerated and strangulated groin hernias [2, 3, 10–13].

The main issues regarding the emergent laparoscopic treatment of complicated inguinocrural hernias are:

1. Type of laparoscopic approach: transabdominal preperitoneal inguinal hernia repair (TAPP) or total extraperitoneal inguinal hernia repair (TEP);
2. Bowel resection;
3. Laparoscopic approach in pediatric patients;
4. Advantages, disadvantages and contraindications.

8.2.1 TAPP

The TAPP procedure may be proposed for the emergency treatment of inguinocrural incarcerated hernias, allowing not only hernia correction, but also visual control and the concomitant treatment of the herniated structures. Visceral vitality is easily established and monitored during laparoscopy: the time dedicated to the hernia repair is an acceptable observation time for the detection of irreversible bowel ischemic damage [2, 5, 10–12]. The use of the TAPP technique facilitates inspection of the contralateral inguinal region and discovery of unsuspected bilateral hernias [14]. However the TAPP approach increases the risk of injury to the abdominal viscera [12, 13].

8.2.1.1 Technical Details

The first step in the TAPP procedure consists of the exploration of the

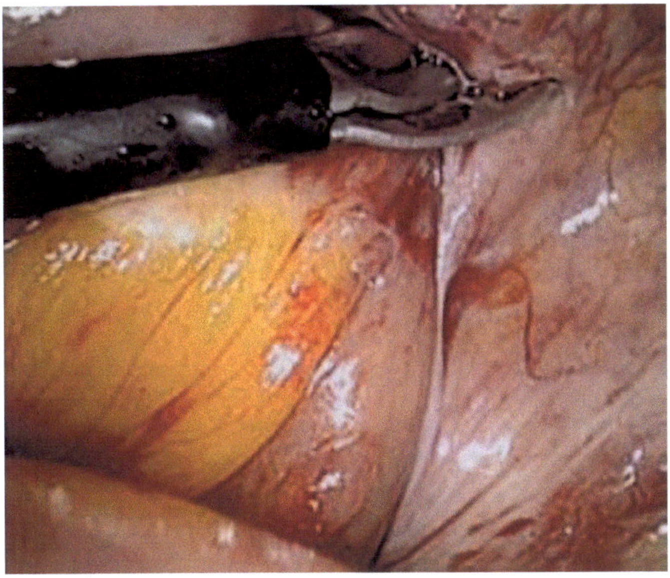

Fig. 8.1 Laparoscopic view of the incarcerated indirect inguinal hernia: reduction of the content obtained by a ventromedial incision of the hernia ring

inguinocrural region and evaluation of the strangulated organs. The second step is reduction of the hernia sac and its contents. Hernia reduction is always obtained by the incision and enlargement of the hernia ring: a ventromedial incision in the case of direct and crural hernias and a ventrolateral incision in the case of indirect hernias (Fig. 8.1). These measures prevent injuries to femoral and epigastric vessels and spermatic cord. After enlargement of the hernia ring, the strangulated bowel is brought into the peritoneal cavity by gentle traction applied to the nondistended loop. The incision of the parietal peritoneum allows reduction of the hernia sac, preparation of Cooper's ligament and parietalization of the cord [10, 11].

8.2.2 TEP

The TEP approach is feasible for the treatment of acutely incarcerated inguinal hernias, however, very precise knowledge of the anatomy involved and total familiarity with the technique are fundamental to undertaking this approach [3, 5]. This method offers the abdominal contents some degree of protection from injury [12] without the possibility of complete visceral control [3].

8.2.2.1 Technical Details

Like the TAPP approach the first step consists of the exploration of the inguinocrural region and evaluation of the strangulated organs. In cases of direct hernia, Cooper's ligament and femoral canal usually are obscured by the contents of the defect. It is important also in this approach to enlarge the opening of the defect to allow safe dissection of the contents. This releasing incision should be made at the anteromedial aspect of the defect to avoid injury to the epigastric or iliac vessels. When an indirect hernia is incarcerated, as with some large sliding or giant scrotal hernias, the large indirect sac invades the posterior inguinal wall, causing a bulge inward in the medial fossa. In these cases, the approach to the internal ring must start with identification of the epigastric vessels. Because the deferent cord is adjacent to the epigastric vessels and the loops toward the space of Retzius, dissection should be started in the anterolateral aspect of the deep internal ring. Additional steps will help: the epigastric vessels may be divided to allow easier dissection of the sac. The deep internal ring is divided anteriorly at the 12 o'clock position toward the external ring, facilitating dissection of the indirect sac. In cases of incarcerated crural hernias, the dissection is performed along the superomedial and inferomedial aspects of the femoral canal to avoid injury to the external iliac and femoral vessels. The sac is reduced by traction and countertraction [3].

The transabdominal approach may be superior in incarcerated and strangulated inguinal hernia with regard to reduction and evaluation of the sac content.

8.2.3 Bowel Resection

Bowel resection can be undertaken as a totally laparoscopic procedure or it can be laparoscopically guided by a minilaparotomy above the area where the non-viable bowel has been laparoscopically located [2]. The resective time is thus shortened compared to a total laparoscopic resective procedure. The visceral manipulation and resection has to be performed only after the closure of the parietal peritoneum at the conclusion of the hernioplasty, thus reducing potential infections of the hernia mesh [11].

The hernia defect is repaired with mesh when there is a very low risk of infection. In cases in which infection risks are high (e.g. ischemic bowel, perforation, presence of pus etc), it is preferable not to place the mesh or, alternatively, a new biologic tissue graft is used to repair these complicated hernia defects [15].

8.2.4 Pediatric Patients

Many hour studies described the safety and effectiveness of laparoscopy in the treatment of inguinal hernia in children. This approach has been recently used in repairing incarcerated inguinal hernias: it is safe, avoids the difficult dissection of an edematous sac in the groin, allows inspection of the reduced hernia content and permits the repair of a contralateral patent processus vaginalis if present and the hospital stay is short [16, 17].

8.2.4.1 Technical Details

First, the herniated structures such as greater omentum, intestinal loops, appendix or ovaries need to be reduced. A mesh is not utilized; the sac is closed with a 4/0 nonabsorbable suture. The last step of the procedure is to reduce the diameter of internal inguinal ring by positioning 1 or 2 separate sutures between the conjoined tendon and the crural arch [16, 17].

8.2.5 Advantages and Disadvantages

Laparoscopic hernia repair, in particular TAPP in emergent conditions, offers real advantages, including the assessment of the vitality of incarcerated organs and the exploration of additional intra-abdominal complications. Moreover, the use of the TAPP technique facilitates inspection of the contralateral inguinal region and discovery of unsuspected bilateral hernias [2, 5, 11].

TEP is not recommended by many authors because it is difficult in cases of massive hernias, it does not allow further control of the reduced viability of the loop in the abdomen is not possible and laparoscopic or laparo-assisted resection [2, 3, 5, 12].

Nonetheless, the rates of complication, recurrence, and hospital stay are very close to the rates documented in open repair for strangulated/incarcerated hernias. This approach is feasible and safe, taking into consideration the knowledge of anatomy and expertise needed in dissecting and reducing the sac [2, 11]. In fact, the learning curve is relatively long: laparoscopic inguinal hernia repair is a difficult technique. If traditional inguinal repair is one of the first actions being proposed to the young surgeon, laparoscopic surgery is considered an advanced procedure that is given only after adequate experience [11].

Abdominal distension, as described for ileal obstruction in general, is the major cause of conversion. Conversion should not be viewed as a failure, but rather a necessary step in the optimal management of these patients [18].

We believe all patients evaluated as being operative candidates in the setting of acute small bowel obstruction should initially undergo the laparoscopic procedure. In fact, this approach is characterized by a high success rate and efficient operation. Therefore, patients will benefit from short operative times, fewer wound complications, quicker recovery, shorter hospital stay and less pain.

8.2.6 Contraindications

All patients potentially can be operated on; the only contraindications are related to anesthesia. Previous pelvic surgery, preoperative clinical signs of strangulation and perforation or hernia dimensional criteria are relative contraindications, depending on the surgeon's ability [5, 10, 11].

8.2.7 Hernia Sac Laparoscopy: Another Opportunity during the Traditional Inguinal Approach

In cases with a spontaneous reduction of the herniated structures, especially when a hemorrhagic fluid is present in the sac, intra-abdominal exploration is mandatory to definitively assess its viability. The 15–20% incidence of reduced gangrenous bowel reported in the literature implies that the proper recognition of intestinal ischemia owing to strangulation is critically important.

Hernia sac laparoscopy is an established safe procedure and allows for an accurate exploration of bowel viability. It can reduce the number of unnecessary laparotomies. Particularly in high-risk patients it may produce a decrease in major morbidity [13, 19].

8.2.7.1 Technical Details

A 10 mm trocar is inserted through the internal inguinal ring, a tight purse-string suture is placed on the hernia sac and a 10 mm optic is positioned for the inspection of the incarcerated structure and its viability. When detecting gangrenous herniated structures, additional ports may be inserted to reset them. Alternatively an open minilaparotomy is performed [13].

8.3 Incarcerated Ventral and Incisional Hernia

Incisional hernia is a common complication in abdominal surgery. It is reported to develop in 3–29% of laparotomic incisions, with an increasing incidence in patients who develop wound infections or other forms of wound complications. Complications such as incarceration or strangulation may occur in 5% of cases [20, 21]. Urgent operations may be required in 5–13% of incarcerated abdominal wall hernias cases and intestinal resections may be required in 10–15% [22].

Emergent laparoscopic treatment of incarcerated incisional hernias seems to be one of the most interesting and debated topics [20]. Apart from case reports and few case series, the role of laparoscopic treatment of ventral/incisional hernias in emergent situations for strangulation and/or incarceration has not been established to date, due to the reluctance to use this approach in such situations [20–23].

In these instances a traditional open approach is preferred without placing a mesh in most cases, aiming at the resolution of the life-threatening condition and delaying definitive repair. On the other hand there is available evidence that demonstrates the superiority of the laparoscopic approach in various abdominal emergencies [23].

In 2006 the Consensus Conference of the European Association of Endoscopic Surgery (EAES) developed evidence-based recommendations for the laparoscopic treatment of abdominal emergencies: it was stated that the open approach remains the standard treatment for incarcerated hernia, although laparoscopic surgery may be considered in carefully selected patients and restricted to surgeons with maximum expertise in this field [24]. In 2010, an Italian Consensus Conference of the main National Scientific Societies (SIC-Società Italiana di Chirurgia, ACOI-Associazione Chirurghi Ospedalieri Italiani, SICE-Società Italiana di Chirurgia Endoscopica and EHS-Italian Chapter of European Hernia Society) on laparoscopic treatment of ventral and incisional hernia underlined that, in emergent cases, the incidence of intra-postoperative complications and recurrences is the same as in elective cases [25]. Good experience in emergency surgery and in laparoscopic repair of the abdominal wall in elective patients is always strictly required. Between the two Consensus Conferences more numerous case series [20, 21, 26] have been published.

The main issues regarding the emergent laparoscopic treatment of complicated ventral and incisional hernias are:

1. patient selection;
2. details of surgical technique;
3. surgical experience;
4. use of biological meshes.

8.3.1 Patient Selection Criteria

- *Absence of conspicuous abdominal distension* that precludes entry into the peritoneal cavity and limits adequate working space. Some studies report that a small bowel diameter exceeding 4 cm, at a preoperative abdominal x-ray, and a late operation (>24 hours post-onset, >6 hours post hospital admission) predict an increased risk of conversion [23, 27–29];
- Some authors introduce the *number (>4) of previous laparotomies* as a predictive factor of conversion [23]. However, not only the number but also the type of previous procedure and the location of the surgical scars are very important. As far as adhesiolysis is concerned, one surgical xiphoid-pubic scar following an abdominal trauma or massive peritonitis will often give rise to more difficulties than three scars (e.g. in the right subcostal area, in the hypogastrium and in the right iliac region) resulting from elective and uncomplicated surgery [29];
- *Absence of peritonitis* with the need for bowel resection and bowel handling in a highly inflamed environment [30] and *absence of clinical signs of intestinal ischemia;*
- *Absence of high septic risk situations,* such as concomitant execution of contaminated abdominal procedures or the presence of contaminated skin lesions or enterocutaneous fistulae [20];
- *Absence of major defects* with loss of domain or hernias that do not allow the laparoscopic approach with adequate over-lap [20];
- *Absence of hemodynamic instability and severe co-morbid conditions such as heart and lung diseases that preclude the use of pneumoperitoneum* [30];
- *Morbid obesity* [31], *old age and debilitation* are not considered contraindications to laparoscopy [21, 28, 32].

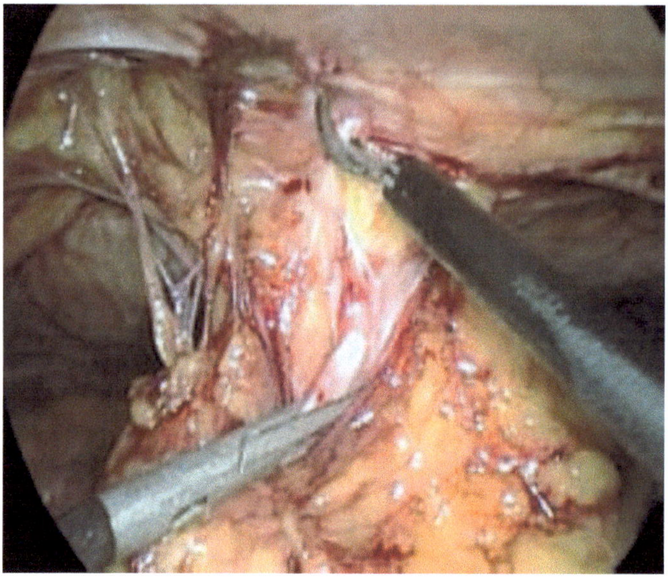

Fig. 8.2 Laparoscopic view of the incarcerated incisional hernia of the middle line: reduction of the intestinal contents with enlargement of the hernia port using careful incision of the fascia at the edge of the hernia ring

8.3.2 Details of Surgical Technique

When an incisional hernia is found to be the cause of obstruction, all incarcerated or strangulated intestinal contents are reduced back into the abdominal cavity and inspected for viability [27]. The herniated structure is reduced by a combination of manual external pressure, internal traction, and adhesiolysis.

As in open surgery, traction and counter-traction are the key elements for a successful procedure: with adequate traction and counter-traction, it is possible to identify the avascular plane of dissection [21, 27, 28, 30, 33, 34].

The best way to release the bowel is by enlargement of the hernia port using careful incision of the fascia at the edge of the hernia ring. The use of an atraumatic grasper is mandatory, thus avoiding the use of scissor with cautery capability close to the bowel loops (Fig. 8.2). The next step is similar to the elective treatment: positioning of intraperitoneal mesh fixed with staples.

The crucial part of the laparoscopic intervention is adhesiolysis because it may lead to bowel perforation [20]. Most series reveal no difference between open and laparoscopic groups with respect to iatrogenic injuries to the bowel. In general, iatrogenic injuries were more likely with dense and extensive adhesions [34]. Two bowel injury mechanisms have been described: direct trauma by scissor with no intraoperative recognition and an indirect lesion due to energy source with subsequent necrosis causing the perforation [29].

The need to perform proper adhesiolysis in order to adequately identify the hernia defect allowing the placing of the mesh is crucial [20]; this is particularly important in the emergency setting due to the bowel distention of the incarcerated bowel loops, associated with vascular compromise with possible development of necrosis and contaminated effusion and the impossibility of performing adequate preoperative bowel cleaning [30].

The incidence of recognized enterotomies varies from 6 to 14.3%; the management of this condition is somewhat controversial: in many centers the hernia procedure is terminated and the injury is repaired either laparoscopically or by conversion to open technique and the hernia repair deferred [35]. Most recently some authors have reported the feasibility of repairing the enterotomy laparoscopically and completing the procedure with the application of mesh in cases where the injury is not associated with a large amount of spillage of intestinal structures [15, 25, 28]. We suggest repairing the lesions laparoscopically if the iatrogenic lesion involves the small bowel, without fecal contamination of the abdomen, and to proceed in positioning the mesh. If the lesion involves the colon or if there is fecal contamination, we prefer to suture the perforation, clean the abdomen and place the mesh during a second operation [21, 27, 33].

Moreover, surgeons must be very careful and check the bowel at the end of the procedure to avoid any undiscovered lesion which in the postoperative period can cause peritonitis. Peritonitis is the major complication that occurs in up to 6% of patients and can lead to fatal consequences involving a 0.3% mortality [26]. This implies a strict early postoperative follow-up to identify suspicious symptoms and signs like fever, leukocytosis, increasing abdominal pain to establish a correct diagnosis and an early reoperation. Some authors identified three categories of patients with high risk of visceral injury [23]:

1. hernias with multiple bowel loops;
2. previous recent repair with polypropylene mesh;
3. previous episodes of severe peritonitis.

In the presence of incarceration under these circumstances, laparoscopy can still be attempted. However, if release of the incarcerated bowel or release of the bowel adhering to the peritoneum around the herniation cannot be performed safely, conversion to open repair must be initiated [28, 34].

The reasons for conversion are [15, 21, 27, 28, 30, 34]:

1. reduced working space because of intestinal distension;
2. dense adhesions;
3. iatrogenic perforation;
4. bowel necrosis.

Iatrogenic perforation and bowel necrosis are relative reasons because they can be managed laparoscopically [27]. Conversion does not equal failure, but simply the necessary sequence of events in the optimal management of these patients [34].

8.3.3 Surgical Experience

In several studies on laparoscopic repair in emergent situations, the authors mention *learning curves* and *experienced surgeon* without defining them evenly. Studies concerning elective surgery suggest that the incidence of major complications such as a missed enterotomy and mortality tend to decrease as the surgeon's experience increases after at least 50 cases [26, 33, 36]. In particular, in 1998, Voitk [18] introduced the concept of previous basic laparoscopic experience, although in a different field: elective laparoscopic inguinal hernia repair requires a learning curve with 50 operations for surgeons *already experienced in laparoscopic cholecystectomy* and open inguinal hernia surgery. Neither seems to have significant influence on clinical outcomes, although improved experience was reflected in improved operation time, conversion rate, and hospital stay [37].

However, this type of surgery requires experience in both laparotomic and laparoscopic emergency surgery, as well as comprehensive experience in elective laparoscopic repair techniques. It is not possible to define clinical competence because of too many variables: experience in previous different operations, high/low volume surgeon and center.

8.3.4 Risk of Infection of the Mesh and Use of Biological Meshes

The introduction of such materials in clinical practice has provided a new prospective for abdominal wall defect repair in a contaminated surgical field [38]. Several authors have suggested the use of biomaterial in laparoscopic emergency hernia repair with good results in terms of recurrence rate and wound infection [39, 40]. There are no comparative trials evaluating each of the commercially available biological mesh products and their application in laparoscopic repair of potentially contaminated ventral hernias. Further studies are still required to establish the efficacy of biological mesh in laparoscopic repair in potentially contaminated fields.

In conclusion, laparoscopic treatment of incarcerated hernias seems to be effective even in emergency situations. It may have further advantages over the open technique, especially those related to the minimally invasive nature of the procedure, such as less pain and fewer infections, which lead to shorter hospital stay, quicker return to normal activities and lower cost for the hospital and healthcare system. The contraindications are massive bowel distention and the presence of contamination of the abdominal cavity. An accurate control of the intestinal loops should be performed at the end of the procedure to confirm the absence of any injuries to avoid complications; however, if adhesiolysis or the release of the incarcerated bowel cannot be performed safely, the procedure should be converted early.

References

1. Ghezzi TL, Moschetti L, Corleta OC et al (2010) Analysis of the videolaparoscopy potentiality in the surgical treatment of the bowel obstruction. Arq Gastroenterol 47:148-151

2. Deeba S, Purkayastha S, Paraskevas P et al (2009) Laparoscopic approach to incarcerated and strangulated inguinal hernias. JSLS 13:327-331
3. Ferzli G, Shapiro K, Chaudry G, Patel S (2004) Laparoscopic extraperitoneal approach to acutely incarcerated inguinal hernia. Surg Endosc 18:228-231
4. Schultz L, Graber J, Pietrafitta J, Hickok D (1990) Laser laparoscopic herniorraphy: a clinical trial preliminary results. J Laparoendosc Surg 1:41-45
5. Hoffman A, Leshem E, Zmora O et al (2010) The combined laparoscopic approach for the treatment of incarcerated inguinal hernia. Surg Endosc 24:1815-1818
6. McCormack K, Scott NW, Go PM et al (2003) Laparoscopic techniques versus open techniques for inguinal hernia repair. Cochrane Database Syst Rev 1: CD001785
7. Anadol ZA, Ersoy E, Taner F, Tekin E (2004) Outcome and cost comparison of laparoscopic transabdominal preperitoneal hernia repair versus open Lichtenstein technique. J Laparoendosc Adv Surg Tech A 14:159-163
8. Morrison JE, Jacobs VR (2008) Laparoscopic preperitoneal inguinal hernia repair using preformed polyester mesh without fixation prospective study with 1-year follow up results in a rural setting. Surg Laparosc Endosc Percutan Tech 18:33-39
9. Watson SD, Saye W, Hollier PA (1993) Combined laparoscopic incarcerated herniorrhaphy and small bowel resection. Surg Laparosc Endosc 3:106-108
10. Rebuffat C, Galli A, Scalambra MS, Balsamo F (2006) Laparoscopic repair of strangulated hernias. Surg Endosc 20:131-134
11. Legnani GL, Rasini M, Pastori S, Sarli D (2008) Laparoscopic trans-peritoneal hernioplasty (TAPP) for the acute management of strangulated inguino-crural hernias: a report of nine cases. Hernia 12:185-188
12. Freundlich RE, Hawes LT, Weldon SA, Brunicardi FC (2011) Laparoscopic repair of an incarcerated right indirect sliding inguinal hernia involving a retroperitoneal ileum. Hernia 15:225-227
13. Sgourakis G, Radtke A, Sotiropoulos GC et al (2009) Assessment of strangulated content of the spontaneously reduced inguinal hernia via hernia sac laparoscopy. Preliminary results of a prospective randomized study. Surg Laparosc Endosc Percutan Tech 19:133-137
14. Davis CJ, Arregui MF (2003) Laparoscopic repair for groin hernias. Surg Clin N Am 83:1141-1161
15. Grafen FC, Neuhaus V, Schob O, Turina M (2010) Management of acute small bowel obstruction from intestinal adhesions: indications for laparoscopic surgery in a community teaching hospital. Langenbecks Arch Surg 395:57-63
16. Kaya M, Huckstedt T, Schier F (2006) Laparoscopic approach to incarcerated inguinal hernia in children. J Pediatr Surg 41:567-569
17. Esposito C, Montinaro L, Alicchio F et al (2009) Technical standardization of laparoscopic herniorrhaphy in pediatric patients. World J Surg 33: 846-850
18. Voitk AJ (1998) The learning curve in laparoscopic inguinal hernia repair for the community general surgeon. Can J Surg 41:446-450.
19. Koivusalo A, Pakarinem MP, Rintala RJ (2007) Laparoscopic herniorrhaphy after manual reduction of incarcerated inguinal hernia. Surg Endosc 21:2147-2149
20. Olmi S, Cesana G, Eba L, Croce E (2009) Emergency laparoscopic treatment of acute incarcerated incisional hernia. Hernia 3:605-608
21. Shah RH, Sharma A, Khullar R et al (2008) Laparoscopic repair of incarcerated ventral abdominal wall hernia. Hernia 12:457-463
22. Derici H, Unalp HR, Bozdag AD et al (2007) Factors affecting morbidity and mortality in incarcerated abdominal wall hernias. Hernia 11:341-346
23. Landau O, Kyzer S (2004) Emergent laparoscopic repair of incarcerated incisional and ventral hernia. Surg Endosc 18:1374-1376
24. Sauerland S, Agresta F, Bergamaschi R et al (2006) Laparoscopy for abdominal emergencies: evidence-based guidelines of the European Association for Endoscopic Surgery. Surg Endosc 20:14-29
25. Il trattamento laparoscopico del laparocele. Prima Consensus Conference Italiana. Allegato

al n. 22 del 8-14 Giugno 2010. Il Sole 24 ore. Sanità 5-41.
26. Piccoli M, Ferronato M, Morici R et al (2008) Emergency laparoscopic repair of complicated ventral and incisional hernias. Updates Surg 2:227-235
27. Franklin ME, Gonzalez JJ, Miter DB et al (2004) Laparoscopic diagnosis and treatment of intestinal obstruction. Surg Endosc 18:26-30
28. Kirshtein B, Roy-Shapira A, Lantsberg L et al (2005) Laparoscopic management of acute small bowel obstruction. Surg Endosc 19:464-467
29. Piccoli M, Marchi D, Abati G, Melotti G (2008) Laparoscopic approach in intestinal obstructions: indications, techniques, advantages and constraints. In: Sartelli M, Catena F (eds) Emergency surgery manual. Alpes, Rome pp 227-238
30. Szomstein S, Lo Menzo E, Simpfendorfer C et al (2006) Laparoscopic lysis of adhesions. World J Surg 30:535-540
31. Raftopoulos I, Courcoulas AP (2007) Outcome of laparoscopic ventral hernia repair in morbidity obese patients with a body mass index exceeding 35 kg/m2. Surg Endosc 21:2293-2297
32. Carlson MA, Frantzides CT, Shostrom VK, Laguna LE (2008) Minimally invasive ventral herniorrhaphy: an analysis of 6,266 published cases. Hernia 12:9-22
33. Sharma A, Mehrotra M, Khullar R et al (2008) Limited-conversion technique: a safe and viable alternative to conversion in laparoscopic ventral/incisional hernia repair. Hernia 12:367-371
34. Lujan HJ, Oren A, Plasencia G et al (2006) Laparoscopic management as the initial treatment of acute small bowel obstruction. JSLS 10:466-472
35. Assalia A, Gagner M, Shein M (eds) (2006) Controversies in laparoscopic surgery. Springer, New York
36. Salameh JR, Sweeney JF, Graviss EAet al (2006) Laparoscopic ventral hernia repair during the learning curve. Hernia 6:182-187
37. Neo EL, Zingg U, Devitt PG et al (2010) Learning curve for laparoscopic repair of very large hiatal hernia. Surg Endosc 7:1461-1468
38. Campanelli G, Catena F, Ansaloni L (2008) Prosthetic abdominal wall hernia repair in emergency surgery: from polypropylene to biological meshes. World J Emergency Surg 3:33
39. Parra MW, Rodas EB, Niravel AA (2010) Laparoscopic repair of potentially contaminated abdominal ventral hernias using a xenograft: a case series. Hernia 11:687-687
40. Franklin ME JR, Trevino JM, Portollo G et al (2008) The use of porcine small intestinal submucosa as a prosthetic material for laparoscopic hernia repair in infected and potentially contaminated fields: long-term follow up. Surg Endosc 22:1941-1946

Suggested Readings

Sauerland S, Agresta F, Bergamaschi R, Borzellino G, Budzynski A, Champault G, Fingerhut A, Isla A, Johansson M, Lundorff P (2006) Laparoscopy for abdominal emergencies. Evidence-based guidelines of the European Association for Endoscopic Surgery. Surg Endosc 20:14–29

Agresta F, Ansaloni L, Baiocchi L, Bergamini C, Campanile FB, Carlucci M, Cocorullo G, Corradi A, Franzato B, Lupo M, Mandalà V, Mirabella A, Pernazza G, Piccoli M, Staudacher C, Vettoretto N, Zago M, Lettieri E, Levati A, Pietrini D, Scaglione M, De Masi S, De Placido G, Francucci M, Rasi M, Scaramuzza G, Del Favero AL (2011) Consensus Development Conference of the Società Italiana Chirurgia Endoscopica e nuove tecnologie (SICE); Associazione Chirurghi Ospedalieri Italiani (ACOI); Società Italiana di Chirurgia (SIC); Società Italiana Chirurgia d'Urgenza e Trauma (SICUT), Società Italiana Chirurghi dell'Ospedalità Privata (SICOP) and the European Association for Endoscopic Surgery (EAES). In press

9 Laparoscopy in Acute Mesenteric Ischemia

Gianfranco Cocorullo, Antonino Mirabella, Gaspare Gulotta
and Vincenzo Mandalà

9.1 Introduction

Acute mesenteric ischemia (AMI) is a life-threatening vascular disease which often requires emergent surgical treatment. Early diagnosis and immediate intervention to adequately restore the mesenteric blood flow are mandatory to prevent bowel necrosis and patient death. The underlying cause is varied and the prognosis depends on pathologic findings [1, 2].

Despite the progress in understanding the pathogenesis of mesenteric ischemia and the development of modern treatment modalities, AMI remains a diagnostic challenge for clinicians. Early diagnosis and a prompt effective treatment are essential to improve the clinical outcomes; any delay in the diagnostic process contributes to the continued high mortality rate (59–93%) [2]. Although mesenteric angiography remains the gold standard for the diagnosis of mesenteric ischemia, it is not applicable in many circumstances [3]. The laparoscopic technique has been increasingly used in the diagnosis of underlying diseases, although its implication in the early diagnosis of AMI remains debatable.

The external visualization of the bowel wall alone can dismiss pathologic mucosal and submucosal changes secondary to the ischemic insult in an early stage of AMI [4]. However, in a few circumstances the role of diagnostic laparoscopy might be considered as an adjunct to the process of clinical decision making in the management of patients with mesenteric ischemia. Critically ill patients may represent the target population for whom laparoscopy is worthwhile.

Additionally, diagnostic laparoscopy can be performed at the bedside if the

G. Cocorullo (✉)
General and Emergency Surgery, University of Palermo,
Palermo, Italy

V. Mandalà, *The Role of Laparoscopy in Emergency Abdominal Surgery*,

patient is not transportable. ITU and ICU patients requiring continuous monitoring and support of their vital functions may represent suitable candidates [5].

9.2 Causes

AMI can be divided into occlusive and nonocclusive according to the causative factor. Based on the nature of the obstruction, a further distinction is made within the arterial forms. Moreover, a distinction is also made between venous and arterial occlusions [6].

9.2.1 Arterial Embolism

Arterial emboli are the most frequent cause of AMI and are responsible for approximately 40% to 50% of cases [6]. Most mesenteric emboli originate from a cardiac source. Myocardial ischemia or infarction, atrial tachyarrhythmias, endocarditis, cardiomyopathies, ventricular aneurysms, and valvular disorders are risk factors for the development of mural thrombosis (Table 9.1). Due to its emergence from the aorta at an oblique angle, most visceral arterial emboli preferentially lodge in the superior mesenteric artery (SMA). Whereas 15% of arterial emboli occur at the origin of the SMA, 50% lodge distal to the origin of the middle colic artery, which is the first major branch of the SMA. The onset of symptoms is usually dramatic as a result of the poorly developed collateral circulation [7]. Frequently, the diagnosis of SMA embolism can be made intraoperatively based on the distribution of ischemic bowel. Because most SMA emboli lodge distally to the origin of the middle colic artery, allowing the inferior pancreaticoduodenal branches to be perfused, the proximal jejunum is spared, whereas the rest of the small bowel is ischemic or infarcted.

Table 9.1 Risk factors for the development of mural thrombosis

Risk factors
Cardiovascular diseases (AF, cardiac valvular replacement, endocarditis, heart failure)
PMH: MI, stroke, obliterative arteriopathy of lower limbs
Congenital or acquired hypercoagulable disorders
Age >50
Drug addiction
AIDS
Vasculitis

AF, Atrial Fibrillation; *PMH*, Past Medical History; *MI*, Myocardial Infarction, *AIDS*, Acquired Immune Deficiency Syndrome

9.2.2 Arterial Thrombosis

Acute mesenteric thrombosis accounts for 25% to 30% of all ischemic events. Almost all mesenteric ischemia due to arterial thrombosis occur in the setting of severe atherosclerotic disease, with the most common site near the origin of the SMA. Frequently, patients with this condition can tolerate major visceral arterial obstruction since the slow progressive nature of atherosclerosis allows the development of important collaterals. Bowel ischemia or infarction ensues when the last remaining visceral artery or an important collateral artery occludes. The extent of bowel ischemia or infarction is typically greater than that with embolism, extending from the duodenum to the transverse colon.

9.2.3 Nonocclusive Mesenteric Ischemia

Approximately 20% of patients with mesenteric ischemia have nonocclusive disease. The pathogenesis of nonocclusive mesenteric ischemia (NOMI) is poorly understood but often involves a state of low cardiac output associated with diffuse mesenteric vasoconstriction.

Splanchnic vasoconstriction in response to hypovolemia decreases cardiac output causing hypotension. The resultant lowflow status causes intestinal hypoxia which inevitably leads to bowel necrosis.

Conditions predisposing to NOMI include age older than 50 years, myocardial infarction, congestive heart failure, aortic insufficiency, cardiopulmonary bypass, renal or hepatic disease, and major abdominal or cardiovascular surgery.

However, patients may not have any clear risk factors. Because this condition frequently affects critically ill patients who have considerable comorbidities, the onset may be insidious, and the mortality rates are high.

9.2.4 Mesenteric Venous Thrombosis

Mesenteric venous thrombosis (MVT) is the least common cause of mesenteric ischemia, accounting for up to 10% of AMI [8]. It can be secondary to either intra-abdominal pathologic conditions (such as malignancy, intra-abdominal sepsis or pancreatitis) or the result of primary clotting disorders, with only 10% of cases classified as idiopathic. Mesenteric venous thrombosis is usually segmental, with edema and hemorrhage of the bowel wall and focal sloughing of the mucosa.

Thrombi usually originate in the venous arcades and propagate to involve the arcuate channels. Hemorrhagic infarctions occur when the intramural vessels are occluded. The thrombus is usually palpable in the superior mesenteric vein. Involvement of the inferior mesenteric vein and large bowel is uncommon. The transition from normal to ischemic intestine is more gradual with venous embolism than with arterial embolism or thrombosis (Fig. 9.1).

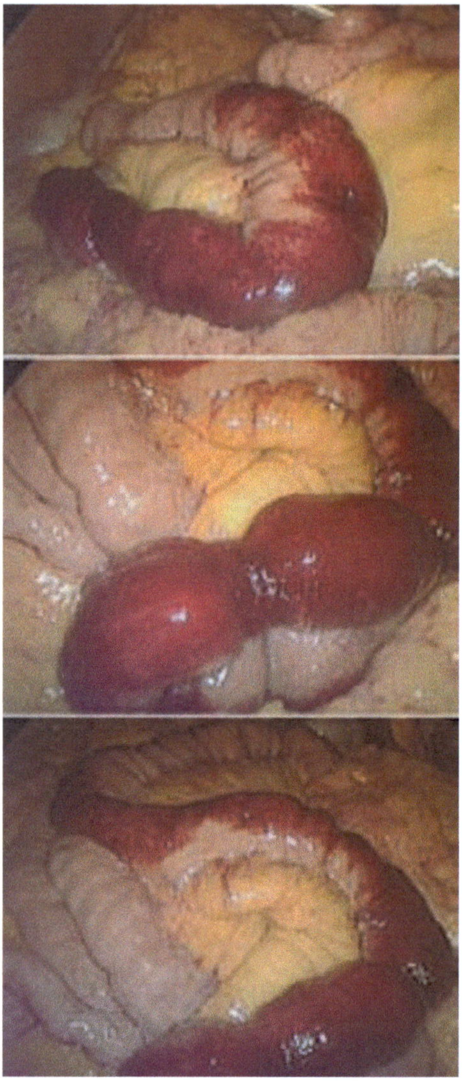

Fig. 9.1 Mesenteric venous infarction in the healing process. Venous stasis is now located only on the portion of the antimesenteric bowel loop. Observation V. Mandalà

9.3 Presentation

Many of the signs and symptoms associated with AMI are common to other intra-abdominal pathologic conditions, such as pancreatitis, acute diverticulitis, small-bowel obstruction, and acute cholecystitis. In addition, the clinical presentation often depends on the underlying pathologic abnormalities. In general, patients with SMA embolism or thrombosis have an acute onset of symptoms and a rapid deterioration in their clinical condition, whereas those with NOMI or MVT have a more gradual onset and a more protracted clinical course.

With SMA embolism, the onset of symptoms is usually dramatic due to lack of collateral circulation, and it manifests as severe and unrelenting abdominal pain, nausea, vomiting and urgent bowel evacuation. Dehydra-tion and excessive fluid loss from third-spacing of fluid lead to mental confusion, tachycardia, tachypnea, and circulatory collapse. Laboratory findings including metabolic acidosis with elevated anion gap and lactate levels, leukocytosis, and hemoconcentration may orientate the clinician towards a diagnosis of AMI.

9.4 Diagnosis

Since AMI may rapidly progress to fatal intestinal infarction, prompt diagnosis and treatment are paramount [1, 9]. A high index of suspicion in the setting of a compatible history and physical examination serves as the cornerstone for early diagnosis of mesenteric ischemia. Survival is approximately 50% when the diagnosis occurs within 24 hours after onset of symptoms, but it drops sharply to 30% or less when diagnosis is delayed. Hemoconcentration, leukocytosis, and metabolic acidosis with high anion gap and lactate concentrations are the most common laboratory abnormalities. High levels of serum amylase, aspartate aminotransferase, lactate dehydrogenase and creatine phosphokinase are frequently observed at presentation, but none is sufficiently sensitive or specific to be diagnostic. Hyperphosphatemia and hyperkalemia are usually late signs and are frequently associated with bowel infarction.

The findings on a plain abdominal radiograph in AMI are also nonspecific. In the early stage of the disease, 25% of patients may have normal findings on abdominal radiography. Characteristic radiographic abnormalities, such as thumbprinting or thickening of bowel loops, occur in less than 40% of patients at presentation. Air in the portal vein is a late finding and is associated with a poor prognosis. In the presence of a high suspicion of AMI the CT scan is the radiologic investigation which provides more accurate and specific details. Several studies have reported a sensitivity of 93.3% and a specificity of 95.9% of CT scan with i.v. contrast [3, 9].

Thickened bowel walls, intramural hematoma, dilated fluid-filled bowel loops, engorgement of mesenteric vessels, pneumatosis, mesenteric or portal venous gas, infarction of other viscera, and arterial or venous thrombus may be seen on CT scan. A further enhancement of the imaging can be obtained with CT angiography which remains, in the absence of a clinical indication for emergency laparotomy, the investigation of choice in suspected AMI. Early angiography has been shown to improve survival rates.

Mesenteric angiography can usually differentiate embolic from thrombotic arterial occlusions. Emboli usually lodge where the artery tapers, which is just after the first major branch of the SMA – the middle colic artery. In contrast, thrombotic disease usually involves the origin of the SMA. Thrombotic cases may be characterized by a complete lack of visualization of SMA. Mesenteric venous thrombosis is characterized by a generalized slowing of arterial flow (up to 20 seconds) in conjunction with lack of opacification of the corresponding mesenteric or portal venous outflow tracts. This is usually segmental, in contrast to NOMI, which is diffuse and shows normal venous runoff. In addition, NOMI characteristically shows narrowing and multiple irregularities of the major SMA tributaries, the *string of sausages* sign [3, 9].

9.4.1 Laparoscopy: an Alternative Diagnostic Tool

Although CT scan has been recognized as the radiologic investigation with the highest sensitivity rate, its employment remains extremely limited in some circumstances [10]. Patients with mesenteric ischemia quite frequently suffer from chronic renal impairment and heart failure which do not allow i.v. contrast. Furthermore, severe dehydration and acidotic status often present in such patients and require time-consuming corrections which can further delay the appropriate treatment. Unfortunately the delay can lead to a late diagnosis of AMI by which time bowel changes might have already become irreversible. A laparoscopic diagnostic approach should take place as a substitute to other conventional methods.

In addition, in unstable patients requiring intensive care support laparoscopy can be performed at the bedside, which proves extremely important in terms of being less time-consuming and therefore enabling an early diagnosis.

9.4.2 Limits of Laparoscopy in Early Diagnosis of AMI

Emergency laparoscopic procedures can be used to identify and treat several causes of acute abdomen. An increasing use of diagnostic laparoscopy has also been advocated for unclear abdominal findings and for staging of intra-abdominal malignancies.

Against the background of increasing experience in the area of laparoscopic surgery the effectiveness of the use of keyhole surgery in the early diagnosis of AMI is still a controversial issue [4, 10, 11].

The limited application of the laparoscopic technique in this context seems to be related to the poor intraoperative findings at the early stage of the ischemic insult. As it is clearly known, in the early stage of AMI, the primary changes in response to a defected vascular supply affect the inner layers (mucosa and submucosa) of the bowel wall. A laparoscopy performed at this phase may not detect those changes since the inspection of the serosal surface might be normal. The inability to palpate the mesentery to appreciate the presence or the absence of arterial pulsation is another disadvantage of laparoscopy in the early diagnosis of mesenteric ischemia [4, 10–13].

However, other important changes of the ischemic bowel such as edema and congestion of the bowel with patchy hemorrhages, dark peritoneal fluid or patent gangrene can be detected during the laparoscopic inspection of the bowel.

An experimental study performed on pigs suggests additional precautions with the laparoscopic technique in order to enhance the intraoperative findings in the early stage of mesenteric ischemia. The study described the use of ultraviolet light and IV fluorescein dye to identify AMI. The fluorescein enabled the identification of the viable fluorescent tissue against the characteristic darkened silhouette of the ischemic bowel [14, 15].

Another factor limiting the application of laparoscopy is the effect of the pneumoperitoneum on the mesenteric blood flow. A high intra-abdominal pressure may result in a reduced mesenteric blood supply due to a decreased pre-load with a subsequent fall in cardiac output. High intra-abdominal pressure can also directly affect the aorta and its branches. The intra-abdominal pressure should not exceed 10–15 mmHg [12]. Conscious precautions in this direction enable a safe laparoscopic procedure in most cases.

9.5 Treatment

Once the diagnosis of AMI is made, treatment should be initiated without delay. With the exception of NOMI, which requires primary medical treatment, most cases of AMI need surgical intervention to restore blood supply to the bowel.

The presence of peritoneal signs generally indicates bowel infarction rather than ischemia alone and mandates emergency laparotomy. Even in the absence of bowel necrosis surgical intervention is often necessary to avoid irreversible changes in bowel viability.

The resection of the ischemic bowel is the most common surgical procedure in AMI. A satisfactory arterial pulse, a good vascular supply of the section margins and the absence of intra-abdominal sepsis may confidently lead to an immediate bowel anastomosis.

Intra-abdominal contamination, uncertain section margins, and overall poor patient conditions generally contraindicate a bowel anastomosis. In these circumstances the exteriorization of both bowel ends represents a safer surgical procedure.

A small number of patients with occlusive AMI, particularly in the presence of reversible changes, may benefit from other revascularization techniques. Embolectomy, thrombectomy, endarterectomy, or bypass may precede bowel resection in patients with occlusive AMI.

Massively extended gangrene is generally not treated surgically as it will not lead to any significant improvement of the clinical condition [3, 9].

9.5.1 Possible Applications of Laparoscopy

Laparoscopy is a quick and easily applicable procedure. The shorter procedure time is one of its advantages which should not be underestimated when the decision needs to be taken in a short space of time. In patients with severely compromised status, laparoscopy is considered a safe procedure [3].

Acute abdomen on a background of acidotic status may arise from several causes. Laparoscopy should be advocated in those conditions as an essential tool for the differential diagnosis. ITU patients might not be able to sustain surgical trauma and unnecessary laparotomies should be avoided. A large percentage of these laparotomies have negative results or are nontherapeutic, and a negative and nontherapeutic laparotomy can be associated with a morbidity rate as high as 5% to 22% [12]. Several studies [4, 5] have reported that a laparoscopic evaluation can prevent unnecessary laparotomy in 25% to 50% of these types of patients, as well as reduce the mortality rate in critically ill patients. As a very frail group, critically ill patients should be given a chance to avoid major surgical trauma which can be fatal in such poor clinical conditions.

In addition, the possibility of performing a bedside laparoscopy draws a line for a laparoscopic approach in patients requiring continuous hemodynamic and respiratory intensive care support. The advantages of this technique include avoiding the transport of critically ill patients, rapid diagnosis, avoidance of ancillary tests and possibly low cost.

In a retrospective study carried out in the Intensive Care Unit of Texas Endosurgery Institute, Jaramillo et al. [5] reported the usefulness and safety of bedside laparoscopy in 13 years of experience. The study included 13 patients with a mean age of 75.5 years. All patients were under mechanical ventilation and sedated in most cases. The laparoscopy was easily performed by using local anesthesia and administration of i.v. sedation. The pneumoperitoneum was established with a Verres needle and intra-abdominal pressure was maintained at 8–10 mmHg. The mean procedure time was 35 minutes. There was no need of inotrope administration during the procedure. A total of 46% of the patients were diagnosed with mesenteric necrosis and died within 48 hours with no further testing and procedures. Instead 30% of patients had negative laparoscopy, one patient was found with massive fecal contamination and he died the same day. The remaining 15% of patients were found with acute acalculous cholecystitis. No intraoperative complications occurred.

The study mentioned above pointed out the importance of laparoscopy in the differential diagnosis of intra-abdominal conditions. It also suggested that unnecessary laparotomies should be avoided in critically ill patients as further surgical intervention may not be life saving.

Another potential application of laparoscopy in the diagnosis of AMI regards ICU patients. In the early postoperative period after major cardiac surgery using extracorporeal circulation, abdominal complications can have serious consequences with a mortality rate of up to 70%. Early diagnosis and the timely institution of therapy are the most important factors for improving the outcome; however, clinical evaluation of the abdomen is difficult in these patients [5].

A German study carried out in the Department of Surgery at Heidelberg

University reports the accuracy of laparoscopy in detecting abdominal complications after cardiac surgery. The study was performed in 17 patients. In one patient laparoscopy showed no abnormal findings. Six out of 17 patients were found with ischemic right colon whereas five out of 17 were found with massive distension of the large bowel without ischemia on both laparoscopy and laparotomy. Three patients suffered from acute cholecystitis, which was correctly diagnosed by laparoscopy in all cases. In one patient, laparoscopy revealed fibrinous peritonitis without other findings. Open exploration failed to identify the cause of the peritonitis in this patient. Laparoscopy showed no pathologic findings in one patient, but laparotomy then revealed necrotizing pancreatitis confined to the lesser sac. There was one laparoscopy-associated intraoperative complication (6%) in this series [16].

9.5.2 Second-Look

In 1921 Cokkins [17], in describing AMI, reported that *the diagnosis is impossible, the prognosis hopeless and the treatment useless.* In spite of great advances in diagnostic techniques, surgical and non surgical reperfusion and a better supportive intensive care, the mortality rate of AMI still remains high. Several studies report a mortality rate of 59%–93% [4, 11]. Lack of pathognomonic symptoms and its subsequent late diagnosis limit the therapeutic options to bowel resection with or without vascularization. Since the ischemic changes can progress and involve the preserved bowel, the assessment of bowel viability becomes imperative postoperatively. In mesenteric venous thrombosis even after resection of the necrotic bowel and the institution of anticoagulation therapy the process of thrombosis may progress as the thrombus can involve branches distant to the ischemic segment [13].

In 1965 Shaw [18] introduced a second-look laparotomy to overcome the difficulty in assessing the adequacy of bowel resection during surgery. Initially indicated after bowel resection followed by anastomosis or endarterectomy, as well as other vascular procedures such as bypass, a second look nowadays still finds wide application. The awareness of the potential onset of ischemic changes in different segments in fact suggests its use in assessing bowel viability when both ends have been exteriorized.

However, the timing of a second-look procedure is unclear particularly in a patient with anastomosis. Yanar et al. [19] report the data collected after a planned second-look laparoscopy in the management of AMI. In 13 patients, a second-look laparoscopic examination performed 72 h post-operatively revealed normal bowel viability, but in one patient intestinal necrosis was detected. In two of the patients, a third operation was necessary to correct anastomotic leakage. The overall complication rate was 42.8%, and in-hospital mortality rate was 57.1% (n=6) [19].

As the majority of anastomotic leakage occurs on the 3rd to 5th postoperative days, a second-look can contribute to early detection of leakage and prevent peritonitis. Unless earlier intra-abdominal sepsis occurs, a second look operation should be performed within 48–72 h from the first surgical procedure [19].

9.5.3 Laparoscopic Second-Look

In contrast to the limited use of laparoscopy in the early diagnosis of AMI, the technique is becoming increasingly used as a substitute to the traditional surgical second look approach. Although initially described as a traditional open procedure, a second-look laparoscopy seems to have a wider application in selected patients. Since there are no predictive criteria to the progression of bowel ischemia, a laparoscopic second-look could reduce severe unnecessary anesthesiologic and surgical trauma which may prove detrimental in critically ill patients. Unnecessary surgical second-look should be avoided in such circumstances.

A review of the literature from 1994 to date reveals that 19 procedures have been reported to prevent 12 (68%) unnecessary laparotomies [5].

Anadol et al. [22] compared open and laparoscopic *second-look* procedures in patients with mesenteric ischemia. In the first group (n=41), the abdomen was closed and second-look laparotomy was performed in 23 patients. In the second group (n=36), a 10-mm trocar was inserted before closing the abdomen and second-look intervention was performed by a telescope in 23 patients. Sixteen relaparotomies in the first group (70%) revealed nothing and were unnecessary. Two patients (8%) in the laparoscopy group needed repeat resection while 20 patients (87%) were spared from unnecessary laparotomies. The authors concluded that patients with mesenteric ischemia are *ill enough* to deserve the *minimal invasion* spirit of laparoscopic surgery [22].

Second-look laparoscopy is described as a safe method to determine further bowel viability and it is associated with reduced general and access-related risk. The fast progression of the disease and its subsequent devastating bowel changes often require a decision to be taken in a short space of time. Less risk and shorter time required to obtain the necessary information lead most surgeons to consider a laparoscopic approach a valid second-look procedure compared to the traditional laparotomy. In addition, a shorter and lighter anesthesia together with the opportunity of performing the procedure at the bedside contribute to minimizing the risk of clinical deterioration in critically ill patients. Moreover a reduced mortality rate can be achieved by shortening the operative time which means less exposure to a surgical insult [5, 19, 20].

9.6 Conclusions

Acute mesenteric ischemia is an uncommon but severe disease which is always associated with other systemic illnesses contributing to a poor prognosis.

Despite the advances in diagnostic methods the mortality rate remains high. If mesenteric ischemia is clinically suspected, conventional imaging is preferable over diagnostic laparoscopy in defining therapeutic management (GoRC) [10].

Intravenous contrast CT scan and angiography still remain the gold standard for early diagnosis of acute mesenteric ischemia. However, in selected patients where the application of conventional radiologic methods is not feasible, laparoscopy may represent an alternative diagnostic choice.

Undoubtedly, laparoscopy has a relevant diagnostic role in critically ill patients as further exposure to unnecessary surgical trauma may be responsible for the deterioration of their condition and subsequent death. Laparoscopy plays an important role in the diagnosis of nonocclusive mesenteric ischemia (NOMI), since angiography in many circumstances can prove inconclusive and the diagnosis often relies on the appearance of the bowel. An important aspect of laparoscopy regards the possibility of performing the procedure at the bedside if the patient is not transportable and requires intensive care support.

Laparoscopy may be recognized as an important diagnostic tool to assess bowel viability in patients who have undergone cardiac surgery [16]. Due to the disadvantages of the technique, which limits its application to selected patients, laparoscopy still has not been fully recognized in the early diagnosis of AMI. In contrast, interest is increasing in second-look laparoscopies. Several published data in fact suggest a reduced mortality rate by using laparoscopy [21]. Second-look laparoscopy has been repeatedly shown to be a safe alternative to laparotomy. The simplicity and ease of laparoscopy may encourage its wider application to benefit more patients. An increasing use of existing methods such as IV fluorescein and the contribution of new technologic tricks may in the near future see its application in the early diagnosis of AMI.

References

1. Dewitte A, Biais M, Coquin J et al (2011) Diagnosis and management of acute mesenteric ischemia. Ann Fr Anesth Reanim. 2011 30:410-420
2. Haga Y, Odo M, Homma M et al (2009) New prediction rule for mortality in acute mesenteric ischemia. Digestion 80:104-111
3. Menke J (2010) Diagnostic accuracy of multidetector CT in acute mesenteric ischemia: systematic review and meta-analysis. Radiology 256:93-101
4. Zamir G, Reissman P (1998) Diagnostic laparoscopy in mesenteric ischemia. Surg Endosc 12:390-393
5. Jaramillo EJ, Treviño JM, Berghoff KR, Franklin ME Jr (2006) Bedside diagnostic laparoscopy in the intensive care unit: a 13-year experience. JSLS 10:155-159
6. Lock G (2002) Acute mesenteric ischemia: classification, evaluation and therapy. Acta Gastroenterol Belg 65:220-225
7. Luther B, Meyer F, Nowak T et al (2011) Chronically progressive occlusive disease of intestinal arteries - short overview from a vascular surgical perspective. Zentralbl Chir [Epub ahead of print] doi:10.1055/s-0031-1271360
8. Harnik IG, Brandt LJ (2010) Mesenteric venous thrombosis. Vasc Med 15:407-418. Review
9. Wyers MC (2010) Acute mesenteric ischemia: diagnostic approach and surgical treatment. Semin Vasc Surg 23:9-20

10. Sauerland S, Agresta F, Bergamaschi R et al (2006) Laparoscopy for abdominal emergencies. Evidence based guidelines of the European Association for Endoscopic Surgery. Surg Endosc 20:14-29
11. Brandt LJ, Boley SJ (2000) AGA technical review on intestinal ischemia. American Gastrointestinal Association. Gastroenterology 118:954-968
12. Baeshko AA (2000) Laparoscopy in diagnosis of intestinal mesentery acute circulatory disturbance. Khirurgiia (Mosk) 5:18-20
13. Chong AK, So JB, Ti TK (2001) Use of laparoscopy in the management of mesenteric venous thrombosis. Surg Endosc 15:1042
14. Paral J, Ferko A, Plodr M et al (2007) Laparoscopic diagnostics of acute bowel ischemia using ultraviolet light and fluorescein dye: an experimental study. Surg Laparosc Endosc Percutan Tech 17:291-295
15. Páral J, Subrt Z, Lochman P (2009) Peroperative diagnostics of acute bowel ischemia using ultraviolet light and fluorescein dye. Rozhl Chir 88:590-595
16. Hackert T, Kienle P, Weitz J et al (2003) Accuracy of diagnostic laparoscopy for early diagnosis of abdominal complications after cardiac surgery. Surg Endosc 17:1671-1674
17. Cokkins AJ (1961) Intestinal ischemia. Proc R Soc Med 54:354-356
18. Shaw R (1965) The second look after superior mesenteric embolectomy or reconstruction for mesenteric infartion. In: Current surgical management. Saunders, Philadelphia, p. 509
19. Yanar H, Taviloglu K, Ertekin C et al (2007) Planned second-look laparoscopy in the management of acute mesenteric ischemia. World J Gastroenterol 13:3350-3353
20. Yanar Palanivelu C, Rangarajan M, Maheshkumaar GS, Rajan PS (2007) Relaparoscopy in the management of acute abdomen due to localized ischemic bowel: a novel technique—case report. Int J Surg 6:89-91
21. Meng X, Liu L, Jiang H (2010) Indications and procedures for second-look surgery in acute mesenteric ischemia. Surg Today 40:700-705
22. Anadol AZ (2004) Laparoscopic "second-look" in the management of mesenteric ischemia. Surg Laparosc Endosc Percutan Tech 14(4):191-193

Suggested Readings

Sauerland S, Agresta F, Bergamaschi R, Borzellino G, Budzynski A, Champault G, Fingerhut A, Isla A, Johansson M, Lundorff P (2006) Laparoscopy for abdominal emergencies. Evidence-based guidelines of the European Association for Endoscopic Surgery. Surg Endosc 20:14–29

Agresta F, Ansaloni L, Baiocchi L, Bergamini C, Campanile FB, Carlucci M, Cocorullo G, Corradi A, Franzato B, Lupo M, Mandalà V, Mirabella A, Pernazza G, Piccoli M, Staudacher C, Vettoretto N, Zago M, Lettieri E, Levati A, Pietrini D, Scaglione M, De Masi S, De Placido G, Francucci M, Rasi M, Scaramuzza G, Del Favero AL (2011) Consensus Development Conference of the Società Italiana Chirurgia Endoscopica e nuove tecnologie (SICE); Associazione Chirurghi Ospedalieri Italiani (ACOI); Società Italiana di Chirurgia (SIC); Società Italiana Chirurgia d'Urgenza e Trauma (SICUT), Società Italiana Chirurghi dell'Ospedalità Privata (SICOP) and the European Association for Endoscopic Surgery (EAES). In press

Laparoscopic Approach in Gynecologic Emergencies

10

Luciano Casciola, Graziano Ceccarelli and Alberto Patriti

10.1 Introduction

There are situations and emergency conditions of women of reproductive age that a general surgeon might be faced with during his/her practice. While many gynecologists are able to treat appendicitis and perform appendectomies (it is worth remembering that the first laparoscopic appendectomy was performed by the German Gynaecologist Kurt Semm) [1], no experienced general surgeon in his or her career has escaped treating women for gynecologic diseases discovered during surgery performed for suspected appendicitis.

The literature shows that on average expert surgeons make a correct diagnosis for appendicitis in 80% of cases, while young surgeons fail to diagnose it in up to 50% of cases. The percentage of wrong diagnoses increases when dealing with women of reproductive age [2].

The use of laparoscopy, especially in emergency settings, allows surgeons to easily explore the entire abdominal and pelvic cavity [3–7]. In the presence of a clear surgical diagnosis – such as appendicitis – the surgeon must not forget to perform an accurate assessment of the patient's pelvic structures, evaluating the status of the ovaries, uterine tubes and uterus in an attempt to identify possible pathologic findings.

The main gynecologic conditions that may present to the general surgeon in an emergency scenario are pelvic inflammatory disease (PID), ovarian diseases, ectopic pregnancy and acute endometriosis. Another important chapter is chronic pelvic pain (CPP), caused by a number of conditions such as pelvic adhesions. One of the most important consequences of CPP is infertility and intestinal obstruction, which fall in the realm of both the surgeon and the gynecologist.

L. Casciola (✉)
Department of Surgery, Division of General, Minimally Invasive and Robotic Surgery
ASL 3 Umbria, "San Matteo degli Infermi" Hospital
Spoleto (PG), Italy

V. Mandalà, *The Role of Laparoscopy in Emergency Abdominal Surgery*,

10.2 Obstetric and Gynecologic History

In cases of pelvic pain, taking a thorough patient history is mandatory prior to physical examination. The obstetric history is important, particularly if the woman has suffered a late miscarriage, ectopic pregnancy or undergone a Cesarean section. The number and outcome of all pregnancies should be noted together with eventual complications suffered such as abortion, prenatal and postnatal infections (endometritis) and thromboembolism. The gynecologic history should focus on conditions such as pelvic inflammatory and infective processes which are relatively common in women of reproductive age.

Previous surgical interventions such as laparoscopy, hysteroscopy, surgical and medical termination of pregnancy, particularly if recent, have to be taken into careful consideration.

The patient's menstrual history should be checked completely, gathering information relating to her menarche (first menstruation), menstrual cycle pattern and menopausal symptoms. The date of her last menstruation should be recorded as well. The surgeon should enquire as to whether the woman has used any contraceptive methods and their nature.

A delay in the menstruation should lead the surgeon to suspect an ectopic pregnancy, even when the urine pregnancy test result is negative. In such circumstances a serum beta-hCG evaluation would confirm or exclude the diagnosis of a pregnancy. An ectopic pregnancy should also be suspected in the presence of a positive pregnancy test where an intrauterine contraceptive device (IUCD) or oral contraception has been used.

Primary amenorrhea is defined as the absence of a menstrual period in a woman of 16 years of age. Secondary amenorrhea is defined as the cessation of menstruation for at least 6 months or for a period longer than three of her previous cycles. Other irregularities in the menstrual cycle should be recorded.

The average age at which menarche takes place is 12.5 years. In the first 2 years menstruation cycles can be irregular in intensity and length. The menstrual cycle usually lasts approximately 28 days, with a normal range of 23–35 days. Weight, diet, stress, exercise and drugs can all affect the menstrual cycle pattern. The menstrual cycle can be modified by drug therapies. Drugs that may induce amenorrhea are metoclopramide, ulcer healing drugs such as H_2-receptor antagonists (ranitidine, cimetidine), antipsychotics, barbiturates, anxiolytics and steroids. Drugs associated with prolonged periods are non steroidal anti-inflammatory drugs (NSAIDs), parenteral anticoagulants (standard, unfractionated and low molecular weight heparin) and oral anticoagulants (warfarin). Menstrual cycle anomalies can be a sign of systemic diseases such as coagulation, endocrinologic and metabolic disorders.

Vaginal bleeding can be present in newborn girls. Early signs of puberty such as breast development should be sought. Detecting the presence of small follicular cysts through ultrasonography (US) may strengthen the suspicion of an early onset of puberty.

10.3 Clinical Examination and Laboratory Investigations

Clinical examination can confirm or refute a diagnosis suggested by the patient history. Generally a painful abdomen with localized or widespread tenderness, rebound tenderness and, reduced bowel movements should be considered a surgical problem. Urgent hematologic and abnormal ultrasound will help to establish the correct diagnosis. The clinical assessment must always be completed by checking for hernias in the groin or in the site of previous surgery.

Rectal and vaginal examination should not be unduly painful and the reason for performing it must be explained to the patients. The presence of additional medical or paramedical staff during this type of examination is important to ensure that the patient's rights are respected and to prevent any subsequent medicolegal problems. Obtaining patient consent or parental consent of pediatric patients is paramount. The vaginal examination should be avoided in very young patients and in those with virgo intacta.

The physical examination will include palpating the cervix, the uterus and the adnexa. Local tumor, fluid collection and signs of pelvic and peritoneal tenderness will be searched for. Signs of tenderness may indicate the presence of inflammations and infections and suggest peritonitis.

Considering the medicolegal implication, it is advisable to seek gynecologist assistance whenever a gynecologic disease is suspected and if an accurate gynecologic examination has to take place. Unfortunately this may not always be possible, particularly during emergencies, and if this is the case the general surgeons should be able to conduct an accurate gynecologic assessment.

The use of a gynecologic examining couch is preferable to allow correct patient positioning and a good light source is essential. If the examining couch is not available, the patient should be made to lie supine, with the hips and knees flexed and the heels close together. Abduction of the thighs allows adequate access to the external genitalia.

Laboratory investigations should include a full blood count. The red blood cell count and hematocrit will give information on possible anemia. Leukocytosis is always present in cases of infections and inflammations such as salpingitis, PID and pelvic abscesses. It is also often present in the initial stages of an ovarian cyst rupture and in ovarian torsion. Blood cross-matching is advisable before surgery.

Likewise the clotting screen is also necessary in the presence of heavy blood loss or if acute anemia is suspected. The serum human chorionic gonadotropin (beta-hCG) should be urgently tested, particularly in women with irregular menstrual cycles or those using contraception. The serum beta-hCG test should be carried out even when a negative urine pregnancy test result has been obtained, due to a false negative rate of 5%.

Testing for CA-125 is not required in an emergency setting. However it is worth knowing that a raised CA-125 is a specific marker of peritoneal reactions. Levels can be elevated up to one hundred times in endometriosis and pregnancy and a thousand times in ovarian cancer.

10.4 Most Common Gynecologic Emergencies

The most common gynecologic emergencies causing acute pelvic pain are reported below:

1. PID: acute salpingitis, tubo-ovarian abscess;
2. Ectopic pregnancy;
3. Adnexal-ovarian torsion;
4. Ovarian cyst; cyst ruptures (luteal cyst, functional cyst, Mittelschmerz syndrome, endometriomas, cystic teratomas);
5. Endometriosis;
6. Chronic pelvic pathology: chronic appendicitis, endometriosis, pelvic adhesions, Fitz-Hugh-Curtis syndrome;
7. Gynecologic pelvic trauma.

10.4.1 Pelvic Inflammatory Disease: Acute Salpingitis, Tuboovarian Abscess

PID is the term used to describe an inflammatory status of a woman's reproductive organs, often secondary to a sexually transmitted infection of the lower and upper genital tract. The infection can develop in the uterine tubes (salpingitis), ovaries (oophoritis), endometrium (endometritis), the peritoneum surrounding the reproductive organs (peritonitis) or a combination of these. PID can develop mono or bilaterally in the pelvis, but in the former will soon spread widely in the lower pelvis.

Among the most serious complications are tuboovarian abscesses causing permanent damage with the formation of hydrosalpinges and tubal blockage [8, 9]. Infertility is a long-term risk for a patient with a history of PID. A single episode of PID causes tubal damage and consequent infertility in 15–20% of patients with an eight times increased risk of having an ectopic pregnancy. As many as 50% of women will have permanent tubal damage after three episodes of PID [10, 11].

PID mostly affects sexually active women between the ages of 15 and 24 years, and in 30% of cases they are younger than 20 years of age. About two in every 100 women develops PID per year, although this figure may underestimate the real number as many women with PID experience few or no symptoms. Most cases of PID are due to microorganisms transmitted through sexual intercourse. In Western countries *Chlamydia trachomatis* is responsible for 60% of all cases of PID, while *Neisseria gonorrhoeae* accounts for 15%. Mycoplasma and other anaerobic bacteria might also be the cause of PID. About 10% of all PID cases are due to a dual infection with both *C. trachomatis* and *N. gonorrhoeae*. In developing countries tuberculosis, puerperal sepsis and infections following abortion are also important etiological causes [12].

Sometimes the infection that leads to PID may start as a result of bacteria introduced into the vagina or upper genital tract during a surgical intervention for miscarriage, or during uterine instrumentation such as endometrial biopsy, cervical smear test, fitting of an IUCD or investigations to assess the status of tubal patency, such as hysterosalpingography and chromoperturbation at laparoscopy. In other cases the infection is transmitted through contact with pelvic organs that are located close to the site of, for example, appendicitis and diverticulitis.

The symptoms of PID are nonspecific and include pyrexia (often above 38 °C), abdominal guarding, paralytic ileus, nausea, vomiting and oliguria. The pain is often acute and localized in the lower abdominal quadrants and the pelvis. It often radiates towards the back, the sacrum and down to the root and along the legs.

Abdominal and pelvic examination helps to make a diagnosis. The vaginal examination often highlights a pelvic mass in the adnexal areas. Cervical palpation causes acute pain known as cervical excitation. At speculum examination copious and abnormal discharge is often revealed. Bacteriologic testing must be done to make a correct diagnosis and ensure the correct pharmacologic treatment is given. A urinary tract infection might also be associated with PID. Peritonitis may ensue when the infection has spread to the peritoneum. Blood tests will show leukocytosis with high neutrophilia, raised erythrocyte sedimentation rate (ESR) and increased levels of C-reactive protein (CRP). Although laparoscopy could be considered the gold standard investigation for PID, as it allows the targeted collection of intraperitoneal specimens for microbiologic investigation, it fails to highlight macroscopic diseases in 15–30% of cases. On the other hand, laparoscopy helps to exclude other differential diagnoses.

Bacteriological tests of the vaginal, endocervical, and peritoneal secretions should be performed whenever possible to maximize the chances of reaching a definitive diagnosis.

The US evaluation can highlight the presence of pelvic fluid collections and tuboovarian abscesses. A magnetic resonance imaging scan is of limited value in the diagnosis of PID. As there is no specific test for PID, its diagnosis is made through the presence of symptoms and through gynecologic examination. A clinical suspicion of PID has a low sensitivity and specificity with a positive predictive value ranging between 65–90%.

Pharmacologic treatment with a combination of at least two antibiotics must be started immediately. Screening and treatment for sexually transmitted diseases should be advised to the patient's partner. In mild forms of PID an oral antibiotic therapy based on metronidazole and ofloxacin 400 mg, twice a day for 14 consecutive days can be administered. Alternatively, a single intramuscular dose of ceftriaxone 200 mg can be used followed by oral treatment of doxicycline 100 mg for 14 days and metronidazole 400 mg twice per day.

In severe cases of PID hospitalization is necessary and intravenous (IV) antibiotic therapy must be administered for at least 48 hours. The simultaneous use of 2 g of cefoxitin, three times per day and of doxicycline 100 mg twice per day, administered orally or IV, must be followed by at least a 14-day treatment with doxicycline 100 mg and metronidazole 400 mg twice a day. An alternative therapy is the intravenous use of clindamycin 900 mg and gentamycin 1.5 mg per kilogram of weight, three times per day until the fever disappears, followed by 14 days of therapy with metronidazole 400 mg twice per day or clindamycin 450 mg four times per day, both orally.

In some cases, especially when the symptoms do not diminish and when US highlights one or more pelvic abscesses, which occurs in 30–40% of cases, a surgical lavage is required to allow the drainage of the infected collections. At surgery adhesiolysis and excision of necrotic tissue can be performed together with an accurate irrigation and washing of the pelvic cavity [13]. The risk of spreading purulent infective materials in other abdominal areas is always present and could lead to a painful postoperative abscess. In most cases the drainage of a pelvic abscess during PID can be accomplished by laparoscopy or under ultrasound guidance, but in cases of ruptured tuboovarian abscesses surgery is compulsory.

It is important to highlight that the clinical scenario is often confused with that of acute appendicitis. The simultaneous presence of an intrauterine pregnancy excludes the possibility of PID, except when septic abortion occurs.

Lastly, in a woman with suspected PID the laparoscopic approach for the diagnosis has the advantage of facilitating the exclusion of differential diagnoses. The possibility to explore the whole pelvis and abdominal cavity and to collect pathologic material make laparoscopy invaluable for an accurate diagnosis and for establishing the targeted antibiotic therapy [14, 15]. The patient and her partner's follow up is important as PID often recurs. Bacteriologic screening of cervical secretions or of the first midstream morning urine should be repeated 3 months after the therapy is over to screen for *Chlamydia*.

10.4.2 Ectopic Pregnancy

Ectopic pregnancy is the leading cause of pregnancy-related death in the first trimester, and it is a cause of significant morbidity. It is responsible for 10% of maternal deaths.

The implantation of an embryo outside of the uterine cavity is called an ectopic pregnancy. The incidence of an ectopic pregnancy is 1% of all pregnancies and has a high mortality rate of 1 in every 2700 cases in Western countries. In 80–90% of cases the embryo is implanted in the tube ampullary region, and it decreases in order in the isthmic (5–10%), fimbrial (5%) and interstitial (corneal) region (1–2%). Seldom might the pregnancy implant in to the abdomen, ovary and/or cervix (Fig. 10.1).

Any condition that can cause a defective transport of the egg or embryo could potentially cause an ectopic pregnancy. Among the main risk factors for ectopic pregnancies are previous pelvic infections and inflammatory processes (PID, salpingitis, appendicitis or endometriosis), pelvic surgery, tubal surgery (sterilization), a previous ectopic pregnancy, the presence of IUCD, estro-

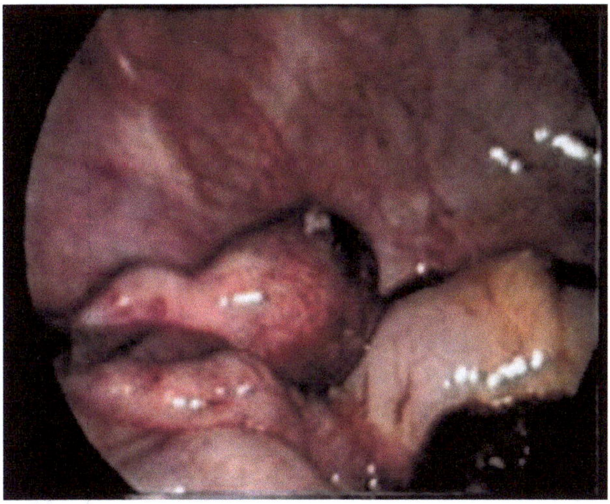

Fig. 10.1 Ectopic pregnancy in the isthmic tubal segment

progestinic therapy and congenital anomalies.

The three main symptoms of ectopic pregnancies, namely, amenorrhea, pelvic pain and uterine bleeding are present simultaneously in about 50% of cases. If hemoperitoneum occurs, then the pain can extend and radiate to the shoulders, mainly the right one due to the subdiaphragmatic irritation of the phrenic nerve. In a high percentage of cases the symptoms are subtle and the pelvic pain can vary in intensity and location. Menstrual delay is often absent in the anamnesis and thus vaginal bleeding can be confused with the menstrual cycle.

The increased awareness of this problem amongst women as well as the advanced diagnostic techniques that use more accurate diagnostic protocols, such as US and laboratory algorithms with the assessment of beta-hCG and plasmatic progesterone, have allowed medical professionals to make a diagnosis much earlier.

The possible consequences of an ectopic pregnancy range from spontaneous abortion, which generally happens in the initial stages, to the pregnancy rupture, often with tubal perforation. The latter is potentially fatal for the patient as it is accompanied by hemorrhage. Such serious complications can either occur gradually with mounting symptoms, or acutely through massive hemorrhage and hemodynamic shock.

The diagnosis is not always straightforward as it may be confused with a spontaneous abortion, salpingitis, appendicitis or ureteral/renal colic. Its diagnosis is made through an accurate collection of previous medical and surgical history, the menstrual history and clinical observation. A menstrual delay, a positive pregnancy test, either urinary or serum beta-hCG levels, and the presence of an empty uterine cavity at US strongly suggest the presence of an ectopic pregnancy. The three typical US signs of ectopic pregnancy, i.e. an empty uterine cavity, adnexal mass and free pelvic fluid, are seldom present in the first 5 weeks of pregnancy.

The diagnostic process in haemodynamically stable patients with a suspected ectopic pregnancy should include the assessment of the serum beta-hCG. A level of 1800 mIU/mL is usually compatible with a visible intrauterine pregnancy by transvaginal ultrasound, while a level of 6000-6500 mIU/mL is necessary for an intrauterine pregnancy to be seen by abdominal route.

10.4.2.1 Treatment Option of an Ectopic Pregnancy

If the patient is hemodynamically stable, a conservative approach can be used. The serum beta-hCG should be repeated 48 hours from the first sample. An increase of the serum beta-hCG to more than 66% in 48 hours is associated in 85% of cases with intrauterine pregnancies, as opposed to 13% of ectopic pregnancies.

Dosing plasmatic progesterone is also useful for the diagnosis of pregnancies in the first 6 weeks. A value lower than 5 ng/mL (16 nmol/L) is always associated with an abortion, both intra- or extrauterine [16]. In an acute pregnancy rupture with the presence of hemoperitoneum an immediate abdominal exploration is required.

The optimal surgical management for a patient with an ectopic pregnancy is dependent on various factors. The patient's age, medical or surgical history and desire for future fertility must be considered together with previous history of an ectopic pregnancy or PID. The size of the pregnancy and the condition of the uterine tube involved should also be evaluated. If the tube involved is ruptured it can rarely be salvaged as the damage occurred is often irreversible. An unruptured ectopic pregnancy in a uterine tube could on the other hand be treated by salpingostomy or salpingotomy (see below), consequently preserving the organ. The condition of the contralateral tube should also be considered as a perfect looking organ might suggest the removal of the affected one. The location of the pregnancy in the tube affects the successful outcome of a conservative surgical approach (Table 10.1).

In an isthmic pregnancy, the endosalpinge is usually damaged and total or partial salpingectomy is preferred over a more conservative approach. On the other hand, a fimbrial pregnancy can be teased out and expressed through the fimbrial end, hence preserving the tube. This conservative approach is often complicated by bleeding, persistent trophoblastic tissue and tubal damage that may predispose to a further ectopic pregnancy.

An interstitial (corneal) pregnancy is a very challenging condition. The pregnancy grows in the segment of the uterine tube that enters the uterus. The surrounding thick myometrial tissue allows for further development of the pregnancy to an advanced gestational age, often into the second trimester. Rupture of such an advanced pregnancy often presents with catastrophic bleeding. The mortality rate of corneal pregnancies is 2% [17]. A ruptured corneal ectopic pregnancy requires an immediate laparotomy and corneal resection. A hysterectomy may be required for intractable bleeding in a severe-

Table 10.1 Conservative procedures for ectopic pregnancy

Salpingotomy
Milking
Tubal washing
Segmental resection
Salpingcctomy
Adnexectomy
Laparoscopic injection of methotrexate or other drug

ly damaged uterus. Laparoscopic corneal resection using local infiltration of vasoconstrictor agents to prevent heavy bleeding can be attempted in a small ectopic pregnancy, if the patient is hemodynamically stable.

Although surgical management of corneal pregnancies is common, the use of conservative medical treatment with methotrexate in an unruptured pregnancy under 10 weeks gestation has been shown to be a safer option, if carried out under strict medical supervision [17].

Adnexectomy and salpingectomy are most frequently adopted when the tube is not amenable to repair and in women who are not interested in preserving fertility. They can be executed through laparotomy or laparoscopy [18]. Salpingectomy is performed if the pregnancy has irremediably damaged the tube, such as in isthmic pregnancies, and where there is uncontrollable bleeding. The patient's hemodynamic condition would need to be considered prior to deciding which type of surgical approach to apply, laparotomy or laparoscopy.

Salpingotomy, partial salpingectomy and salpingostomy are conservative approaches and should be attempted in women wishing to conceive. The type of surgery will depend on the location of the ectopic pregnancy and on the damage that has occurred.

Salpingotomy (where the serosa defect in the uterine tube is closed with fine, non-reactive, interrupted sutures) or salpingostomy (where the serosa defect in the uterine tube is left open so that it can close by secondary intention) have almost equivalent success with regards to future fertility. Both can be carried out when the tube is not overly dilated (some state less than 2.5 cm in diameter) and when the pregnancy is located in the final part of the ampulla or next to the fimbriae.

Electrosurgery can be used to make the incision using an electroscalpel or point diathermy on the anti-mesenteric aspect of the tube, above the swollen area. The length of the incision should be about half that of the swollen area of the tube, and enough to allow for the complete removal of the gestational sac. Before making the incision the area can be infiltrated with 3–5 mL of diluted vasopressin, (1U per 10 mL of normal saline), which gives the advantage of separating the tubal serosa from the muscle layers. The material that has to be removed looks like a blood clot.

Special attention has to be made to adequately treat the trophoblast implantation site to avoid undesired bleeding. The removal has to be careful not to leave parts of the pregnancy remaining and for this aspiration-irrigation can be a useful technique. The incision can be either left open to heal spontaneously as in salpingostomy, or sutured as in salpingotomy by using 2–3 separated, non absorbable sutures 4-0 involving the full thickness of the serous-muscular layers. Alternatively the serosa alone can be sutured. The functionality of the tube seems substantially similar in both treatments [19]. When the ectopic pregnancy takes place in the isthmic region, a partial salpingectomy can be executed and subsequent microsurgical anastomosis of the two end parts can be carried out at a later time once the ectopic pregnancy has resolved. It is important to consider that the surgical conservative treatments have a risk of *retention of trophoblast tissue* ranging from 3–18%. To this end, serial determination of serum beta-hCG following surgery are necessary until the level reaches zero. Conservative surgical treatments have the advantage, compared to salpingectomy [20], of reducing tissue damage and adhesions, thus reducing the risk of recurrences and therefore have a better prognosis for future fertility.

Conservative medical treatment with methotrexate has gained popularity for the treatment of selected cases of ectopic pregnancies. The drug can be used both systemically and locally, directly injected in to the site of pregnancy by laparoscopy or laparotomy. The results in relation to pregnancy resolution and subsequent fertility are good and similar to those of salpingostomy and salpingotomy. The following selection criteria are paramount for the likelihood of success: the absence of hemoperitoneum, a diameter of the intact ectopic pregnancy of less than 3.5 cm at US, the absence of a fetal heart beat during US and a serum beta-hCG of less than 5000 IU/L. In these cases a single 50 mg intramuscular dose of methotrexate per square meter of body surface is associated with 85–94% of successes in pregnancy resolution. Undesired side effects of methotrexate therapy include stomatitis, an increase in transaminases, gastroenteritis, anemia and transitory thrombocytopenia. Patients failing to react to the methotrexate treatment may need to undergo surgery [19].

All the surgical treatments of ectopic pregnancies described above can be carried out through laparoscopic techniques. An essential requirement for this approach is hemodynamic stability and the absence of specific hemocoagulative or anesthetic contraindications. The location and features of the pregnancy may also be a relative contraindication to the laparoscopic approach, such as a pregnancy in the broad ligament, especially if is complicated by a rupture, interstitial (corneal) pregnancies larger than 4 cm and the presence of significant pelvic adhesions. The laparoscopic approach delivers immediate benefits and a reduction in economic disadvantages due to the decreased hospitalization time required and reduced patient morbidity (Table 10.2) [21].

Among the laparoscopic instruments used bipolar electrocoagulation is preferred to monopolar electrocoagulation to safely secure hemostasis in the mesosalpinge prior to sectioning the specimen. Monopolar point diathermy or scalpel allows a more precise incision above the pregnancy and is therefore

Table 10.2 Laparoscopic vs. open treatment of an ectopic pregnancy

Hospital stay	Lower with laparoscopy
Operative time	Lower with laparoscopy
Return to normal activity	Earlier with laparoscopy
Fertility	No difference
Retention of trophoblast	No difference

favored during salpingotomy and salpingostomy. A suction irrigation device is also essential. The ectopic and other specimens must be extracted, with the help of an endoscopic bag through the 10 mm trocar to avoid spreading the trophoblast with high implantation capacity into the abdominal cavity. Finally, the uterine cavity should not be instrumented until the diagnosis is certain. The external manipulation of the uterus through laparoscopic tools is possible and it does not have any effect on a possible intrauterine pregnancy.

10.4.3 Adnexal-Ovarian Torsion

Adnexal torsion is an uncommon cause of pelvic pain and typically involves the ovary and/or uterine tubes. Adnexal torsion is mainly associated with diseases such as ovarian and fimbrial cysts and hydrosalpinges that cause an increased weight and imbalance of the adnexa (Fig. 10.2). The torsion often involves both the tube and the ovary and is more frequent (up to 60%) in the right side (Fig. 10.3) [19]. In 20% of cases it occurs during early pregnancy, probably due to the enlarging luteal cyst and variation in the ovarian density [22]. Previous surgery, in particular tubal sterilization, also increases the risk of adnexal torsion [23].

A sudden onset of acute pelvic pain that may become intermittently worse over a few hours is usually typical. The pain starts unilaterally and might spread all over the pelvis after a few hours. It is often associated with nausea, vomiting, leukocytosis and fever. US, both transabdominal and transvaginal, will help the diagnosis and possibly suggest the need for surgery. At US the ovary will appear enlarged. Color-Doppler if available can highlight a reduction in the vascular flow in the twisted vascular pedicle. About 75% of cases can be managed conservatively.

Immediate surgery will not only confirm the diagnosis but might also improve the prognosis. The laparoscopic approach should be favored as it allows both conservative treatment, by the uncoiling of the coiled pedicle (detorsion) [24, 25], and adnexectomy if necessary. The uncoiling of the coiled pedicle can be followed by a partial or total recovery of the color of the ovary and tube, indicating a restoration of vascular flow. A color ranging from purple-violet to grey-light blue or black means that the adnexa is irreversibly compromised (gangrene) and adnexectomy is the only solution.

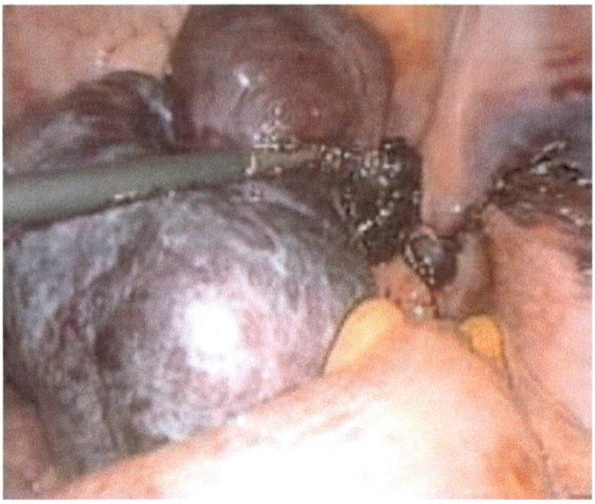

Fig. 10.2 Intraoperative view of adnexal torsion

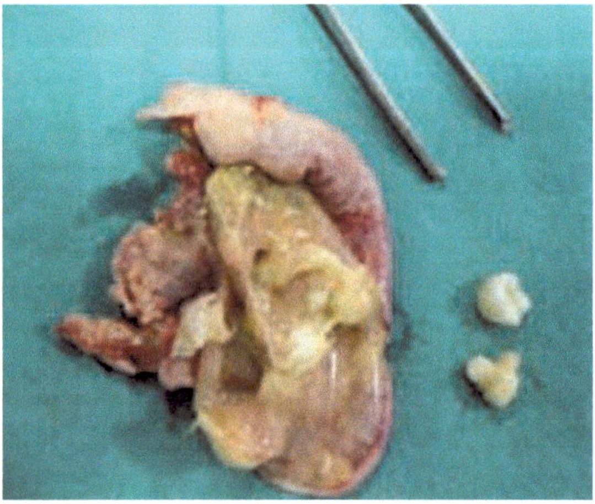

Fig. 10.3 Specimen of a dermoid cyst with differentiated ectodermic tissues

The tools generally used in laparoscopic adnexectomy are monopolar scissors or bipolar dissectors. The modern endoscopic suturing devices make the removal of the torsed pedicle easy and safe. Special attention should be paid to the preliminary identification of the ureter that crosses the bifurcation of the common iliac artery in proximity of the ovarian pedicle and can therefore be easily injured. Large and unsuspicious adnexal cysts might be aspirated prior to their surgical removal to make the tissue manipulation easier. The simple detorsion of the adnexa is sometimes sufficient and no other surgical intervention may be necessary. The success is directly dependent upon the speed at which the diagnosis is made and the intervention is undertaken.

In cases of recurrent torsion or when malformations causing the torsion are present, oophoropexy (stabilization of the adnexa by suture at the pelvic side wall) can be performed to avoid it reoccurring. The shortening of the utero-ovarian ligament by plication and suturing is also used to minimize the risk of further torsion.

10.4.4 Ovarian Cyst; Cyst Ruptures (Luteal Cyst, Functional Cyst, Mittelschmerz Syndrome, Endometriomas, Cystic Teratomas)

Ovarian cysts are usually asymptomatic and are often an incidental finding during investigation or surgery performed for another reason. If symptomatic then lower abdominal pain is the most common symptom, with pain being sharp, intermittent, sudden and severe. A sudden onset of pain may suggest cyst rupture, but more serious etiologies, including adnexal torsion, appendicitis (with or without perforation) and ectopic pregnancy must be considered. Nausea and/or vomiting are associated as non-specific symptoms. Vaginal spotting and irregular menses may occur due to hormonal imbalance in the functional or luteal cysts. Other vital signs associated with ovarian cysts are usually normal or mild fever and tachycardia may be present. Abdominal tenderness is usually unilateral in the lower quadrant and can be severe. Ovarian cysts complicated by adnexal torsion, inflammation, necrosis and hemorrhages may be complicated further by hypovolemic shock. Histologic classification of ovarian cysts according to their frequency shows: functional (follicular or luteal) cysts, endometriomas, cystic teratoma, serous cystadenoma, mucinous cystadenoma and cancerous cystadenoma [19].

Follicular and luteal cysts are normally found in women of reproductive age and are commonly detected during routine surgery or ultrasound. In post-menopausal women ovarian cysts are also common, but the incidence of malignant cysts is greater compared to that of pre-menopausal women. US and cancer markers (CA-125) are very useful for an accurate diagnosis and for surgical planning. In emergency cases the lack of some diagnostic data would initially require conservative treatment.

Follicular cysts are the result of an ovulatory failure with subsequent continuous follicular growth. There can be multiple cysts present in both ovaries. From the ultrasound perspective they appear more often as unilocular with a simple non echogenic structure. They are often incidentallydetected by chance and symptoms are rarely acute unless they are causing ovarian torsion.

Luteal cysts are caused by the lack of regression of the corpus luteum in the late luteal phase of the menstrual cycle. They are generally well vascularized and can bleed during removal or spontaneously, causing hemoperitoneum.

In the differential diagnosis between benign and malignant disease, US plays a major role. Sinister ultrasound signs are septa, solid or complex intracystic components, papillary and fungating growth. Recently the use of color-Doppler has allowed a further characterization of malignant features of ovarian cysts such as low vascular resistance associated with high blood flow.

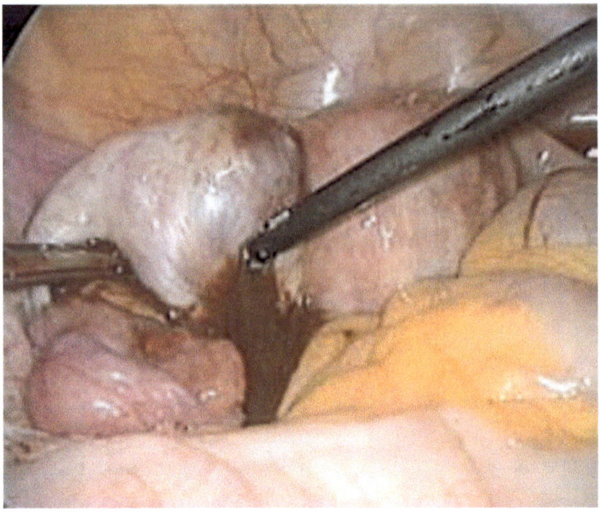

Fig. 10.4 Rupture of an endometriosic cyst

Endometriomas can be recognized by their typical dark color and the chocolate fluid like content (Fig. 10.4). Preservation of the ovary during surgical removal of endometriomas should be attempted, in particular if the patient wishes to conserve her fertility. Surgical treatment options include ovarian cystectomy, which is the intact removal of the cyst, or more often cyst aspiration, cyst wall stripping and oophorectomy. Surgery can be performed either by laparotomy or laparoscopy.

During ovarian cystectomy the ovarian wall can be left in place or sutured with continuous or separated non reactive suture material 3-0 or 4-0. Suturing has however been known to cause periovarian adhesions [19] and should therefore be avoided unless used for hemostatic purposes. Cauterization of the cyst wall to reduce the chance of recurrence must be limited to reduce the damage to the normal ovarian stroma and to its vascularization.

Surgical removal of cystic teratomas carries additional risks compared to other benign ovarian cysts. The material contained in such cysts, if spilled within the abdominal cavity, may give rise to chemical peritonitis. These cysts should be removed intact with the use of intraperitoneal bags accurately inserted and prepared in the abdominal-pelvic cavity to avoid the intracystic material spreading.

Unfortunately in an emergency setting, a complete preoperative work-up of the malignancy potential of the ovarian cyst is seldom possible, yet in situations when the operation can be delayed a serum CA-125 level should always be obtained. It is worth noting that serum CA-125 is still within normal limits in 50% of Stage I ovarian cancers, where the cancer has not yet spread to and beyond the ovarian capsule. During surgery adnexal masses that appeared

Table 10.3 Surgical management of adnexal masses in adolescents

Laparotomy
High suspicion for malignancy
Large cysts
History of or risk factors for abdominopelvic adhesions
Hemodynamically unstable patient – hypovolemia
Significant cardiopulmonary disease
Morbid obesity
Laparoscopy
Minimizing the risks of subsequent infertility resulting from pelvic adhesions
Every effort should be made to conserve ovarian tissue

fixed, irregular or solid, as well as the presence of ascites should raise the suspicion of malignancy (Table 10.3).

10.4.5 Pelvic Endometriosis and Endometriomas

Rokitansky in 1860 described endometriosis as the presence of active endometrial tissue outside the uterine cavity, including tubes, ovaries, pelvic peritoneum, uterosacral ligaments, rectovaginal space, vagina, bladder, intestine, etc.

During menstruation these ectopic tissue areas undergo changes such as edema and bleeding, causing symptoms like acute pelvic pain, dysmenorrhea, dyspareunia, signs of peritoneal irritation, dyschezia, rectal pain and bleeding, each being dependent upon the location of endometriosis. Chronic symptoms with acute bouts of pain are characteristics of endometriosis affecting the ovaries with bleeding, torsion or rupture of an endometrioma.

Apart from the clinical evaluation, diagnosis is helped by transvaginal or transabdominal US and by MRI. Laparoscopy is the gold standard to evaluate pelvic endometriosis as it allows the collection of histologic specimens needed to confirm diagnosis. Deep infiltrating or subperitoneal endometriosis is not always visible at laparoscopy and MRI can therefore be helpful in such conditions. Laboratory investigations are restricted to serum CA-125 which usually increases to values of up to 100–200 IU/mL, but is not useful for the diagnosis. The role of CA-125 is limited to the follow-up of recurrences.

Medical treatment with NSAIDs reduces the production of local prostaglandin, therefore reducing inflammation but more importantly reducing the pain. The medical treatment of endometriosis consists of ceasing ovarian estrogen production. Estroprogestinic preparations are the most useful drugs as they can be used for months if common contraindications such as obesity, breast cancer, smoking and high blood pressure do not exist. The effectiveness of the progestogens medroxyprogesterone acetate and norethisterone are just as good as the common estroprogestinic preparation used for contraception.

Medical treatment by danazol or a GnRH analog are also very effective as a means of stopping ovarian function and estrogen production, but are associated, due to hypo-estrogenization, to undesired side effects including osteoporosis, vaginal dryness, hot flushes and other vasomotor symptoms. The use of danazol or a GnRH analog if protracted for more than 6 months should be associated with an estroprogestinic preparation (contraceptive pill or tibolone) to reduce the menopausal symptoms, osteoporosis and fracture risk. The medical treatment is only effective in minimal endometriosis while moderate and severe forms need to be treated by surgery.

Surgical treatment consists of trying to remove as much endometriotic tissue as possible. It is rare to perform emergency surgery for pelvic pain exclusively due to endometriosis, unless it is secondary to an operation performed for hemoperitoneum due to an ovarian cyst rupture (endometriomas) or for suspected appendicitis. At surgery the removal of endometriosis requires careful manipulation of the organs involved. A careful approach needs to be applied during surgery for endometriosis infiltrating the serosa of the bowel, above the urethra and bladder and above major blood vessels.

Laparoscopy allows a mapping of the disease and the collection of material for histology that will eventually confirm the diagnosis. Surgical staging of endometriosis consists of a scoring to be attributed to each site, localization and extension of the lesion. The most commonly used scoring system suggested by the American Fertility Society helps in the evaluation of patient fertility prognosis [20].

In young women, surgical treatment of ovarian endometriosis must not compromise the reproductive function of the ovary and electrosurgery should be minimally used. The laparoscopic approach, is favored compared to open surgery as it allows clearer visibility and access to the pelvic cavity and reduces the postoperative morbidity and prolonged hospital stay.

It is important to remember that the endometriotic tissue has the capacity to implant and therefore careful peritoneal cavity washing and adequate removal of the surgical specimens should be performed to reduce the risk of distal implant on scars and trocar access points. This peculiarity similar to that of cancerous tissue has been described in a large number of case reports in the scientific literature [26].

10.4.6 Chronic Pelvic Pain: Chronic Appendicitis, Adhesions, Colon-to-Sidewall Adhesions, Fitz-Hugh-Curtis Syndrome

Chronic and recurrent pain in the pelvis or in the right iliac fossa deserves to be dealt with separately. Pain can sometimes be acute and sometimes show subocclusive symptoms which often require periodic hospitalization. In these cases the laboratory and radiologic investigations are essentially normal or minimally significant. These patients are often discharged from hospital without a clear diagnosis.

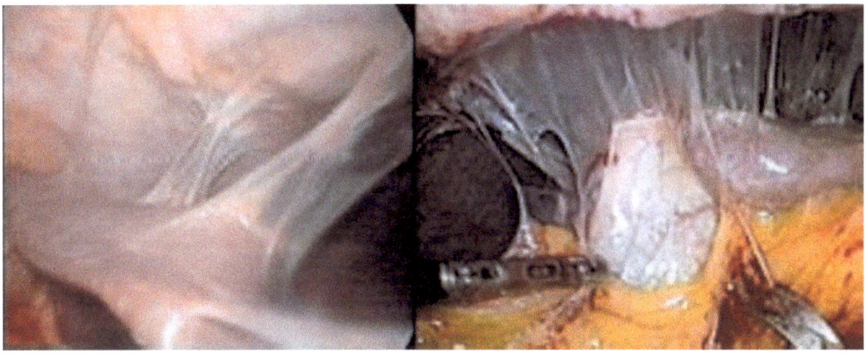

Fig. 10.5 Fitz-Hugh-Curtis syndrome: intraoperative view

Some of those patients will undergo emergency surgery for suspected appendicitis immediately after readmission or after a period of observation if the symptoms do not subside, only to have the suspected diagnosis unconfirmed by the findings at surgery.

The use of the laparoscopic approach in such cases makes the diagnostic evaluation less traumatic and the treatment specifically targeted for the patient's condition. In these forms of undiagnosed pelvic pain where surgery is not only a therapeutic, but also a diagnostic tool, a preoperative strategy should be agreed with the patient. In particular the surgeons should discuss with the patient the surgical steps that will be taken in all possible scenarios. The surgeons must explain the reason for the possible removal of an appendix which is not apparently inflamed, or the surgical steps that would be undertaken should they be confronted with other disease, i.e. adhesions, adnexal pathologies, Meckel diverticulum etc, and obtain the patient's written consent to these treatments.

The greatest advantage of laparoscopy over open surgery is probably the possibility to explore the entire pelvic and abdominal cavity. Acquired or congenital adhesions such as the *colon to sidewall adhesions* (Fig. 10.5) cannot be demonstrated with traditional abdominal incisions such as the McBurney's incision, used for suspected appendicitis. On the other hand, during laparoscopy the set pneumoperitoneum tension between the abdominal wall and the viscera allows visualization and access to these types of adhesions. The increasing use of laparoscopy has demonstrated the so-called *colon to sidewall adhesions* to be present in up to 90% of women with chronic pelvic pain.

Adhesions secondary to surgery are an important cause of infertility [28, 34] and in gynecology the use of anti-adherence barrier solutions have become routine as a preventive measure in such patients [27].

The Fitz-Hugh-Curtis Syndrome is characterized by inflammation of the liver capsule or diaphragm due to ascending PID. Referred to as perihepatitis, it causes the formation of adhesions called *violin string* between the liver capsule and the anterior abdominal wall or diaphragm (Fig. 10.6).

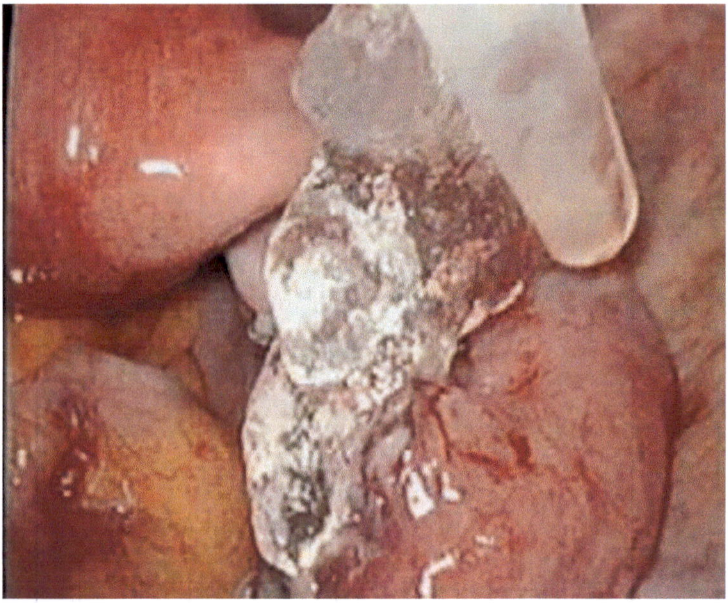

Fig. 10.6 Application of a gel-based anti-adherence barrier solution

Quite often the clinical symptoms resemble those of a biliary colic or cholecystitis, with pain radiating to the right shoulder [29]. It is mainly caused by the *Chlamydia trachomatis* infection and in particular the way the patient reacts to it.

Patients presenting with Fitz-Hugh-Curtis Syndrome often have pelvic adhesions associated with tubal damage and infertility. Yet in about 30% of cases the tubes are apparently not damaged. Fitz-Hugh-Curtis syndrome has been reported to occur following tubal ligation although the pathogenesis appears unclear [30].

10.4.7 Gynecologic Trauma

Many gynecologic traumas (straddle injury, blows to the perineal area, foreign bodies, attempts at abortion, lacerations following childbirth, sexual assault) may involve the pelvic cavity and require surgical exploration and general rules of abdominal trauma management are applicable as well. If the patient is hemodynamically stable, a laparoscopic exploration can be safely carried out, either for diagnostic or therapeutic purposes.

Generally traumas requiring surgery (car accident, gunshot, etc), are complex and involve different cavities (thorax, abdomen, pelvis), therefore they require a multi-disciplinary approach (general surgeon, thoracic surgeon, urologist and gynecologist).

10.5 Laparoscopic Technique

10.5.1 Laparoscopic Instrumentation

Traditional laparoscopic instrumentation is used in pelvic laparoscopy. The most commonly used endoscope for gynecologic endoscopy is the 5 and 10 mm diameter 0º and 30º scope. A suction irrigation system with a suction probe of 5 and 10 mm in diameter is also necessary, especially when dealing with a large hemoperitoneum. Monopolar and bipolar coagulation are routinely used. Bipolar graspers with different jaw shapes and sizes help to control bleeding and are also useful with tissue dissection. Atraumatic graspers are necessary to manipulate the intestine safely. Linear stapling devices with vascular and intestinal cartridges, scissors, endocatch tissue retrieval bag and uterine manipulators are also needed.

10.5.2 Patient Preparation and Abdominal Cavity Access

The patient is positioned supine on the operative bed in a lithotomy position with the hips not fully flexed as this impairs complete access by the surgeon. The space between the legs will allow uterine manipulation. An indwelling Foley catheter should be inserted in the bladder. The catheter can eventually be removed at the end of the procedure or left in situ if the patient has lost a significant amount of blood and is hemodynamically unstable.

A pneumoperitoneum of up to 15–20 mmHg can be induced slowly with a Veress needle into the subumbilical areas in patients at low risk and without abdominal scars, or in the left hypochondrial area (Palmer's point) in high risk patients. An intra-abdominal pressure of about 18–20 mmHg should be reached prior to entering the peritoneal cavity with the primary trocar to reduce the risk of visceral and vascular damage. Once the primary trocar is safely inserted, the intraoperative pressure should not exceed 12–15 mmHg in order to avoid problems with the patient's ventilation. An *open* entry of the peritoneal cavity can also be used in high risk patients. In low risk patients, the first trocar is usually introduced at the level of an umbilical scar. Such access is usually used in almost all diagnostic or interventional procedures as it ensures a good esthetic result for the scar and allows extraction of the surgical specimens.

10.5.3 Trocar Positioning and Abdominal Cavity Exploration

The introduction of secondary (ancillary) trocars takes place under direct vision while trying to avoid any lesions to major vascular structures, e.g. epigastric vessels. Two ancillary ports are usually sufficient. Trocars with the smallest diameter possible should be used, to ensure a lower risk of complications such as bleeding and Richter and small bowel hernias. The positioning of the secondary trocar is chosen in relation to the type of intervention. The secondary trocars are usually positioned in the right and left iliac fossae.

It is good practice to conduct an exploration of the abdominal-pelvic cavity with the endoscope as this enables one to properly assess a suitable position and diameter of the secondary trocars required. Generally, to perform an adequate exploration of the pelvic cavity it would be necessary for the patient to adopt the Trendelenburg position, rotating right or left to assist with the displacement of the bowel from the pelvis.

10.5.4 Drains, Anti-Adherence Barrier Solutions, Trocar Extraction

The insertion of a drain at the end of the surgery, although it may seem unnecessary in the simplest of procedures, can help to ease postoperative pain by reducing intraperitoneal gas. In a complex procedure, the insertion of a drain is almost mandatory as it helps the complete evacuation of the often infected pelvic fluid content. It also allows early detection of postoperative intra-abdominal bleeding. The discomfort that a drain causes to the patient is minimal and it can be removed after 12–24 hours.

The use of anti-adherence barrier solutions such as gels and liquids is advised following intervention where tissue damage and manipulation is extensive and a significant amount of bleeding has occurred. Pelvic adhesions may occur easily following all types of surgery, both open and laparoscopic, however the use of such methods may reduce the adhesion formation as shown in dedicated studies.

In conclusion it is important to stress that one of the golden rules of laparoscopy is the need for meticulous trocar extraction at the end of the intervention to avoid insidious bleeding and recognize the site of potential future hernias. In this regard all portal wounds greater than 10 mm should be closed and various specialized devices are available for this, including J-shaped needles.

10.6 Our Series

In approximately 20 years of minimally invasive surgery practice in a large volume Community Hospital, the laparoscopic approach has played a very important role in the emergency setting. The routine use of laparoscopic exploration allowed us to achieve a good level of confidence in most abdominal and pelvic emergencies. Generally gynecologic emergencies are incidentally encountered during laparoscopy for abdominal pain. Preoperative abdominal and pelvic US is mandatory in young woman, but suffers from low specificity.

Data from the last five years of our series are reported in Table 10.4. A total of 44 women were managed for gynecologic emergencies. A preoperative US

Table 10.4 Our experience of laparoscopic management of gynecologic emergencies: January 2005 – December 2010

Disease	No. cases	Conversion	Associated appendectomy	Associated adhesiolysis	Complications	Mean hospital stay (days)
Complicated adnexal disease (torsion, etc.)	5	-	-	1	-	3.2
Ectopic pregnancy	2	-	-	-	-	3
Pelvic inflammatory disease (salpingitis, tuboovarian abscess)	13	1	5	8	1 persist. pain	3.7
Hemoperitoneum (corpus luteum, follicular cyst, etc.)	11	-	7	-	-	2.5
Pelvic endometriosis (ovarian, bowel, etc.)	13	1	5	7	1 ileus	3.3

examination was always performed, while serum beta-HCG was assayed only in selected cases. In 21% of cases physical examination and imaging were suggestive of acute appendicitis.

When preoperative diagnosis was suggestive of a gynecologic disease (ovarian or adnexal mass, ectopic pregnancy, etc) laparoscopic exploration was confirmatory in 95% of cases and surgery was completed with the minimally invasive approach. The low conversion rate can be imputed to the onging training of the entire team in complex laparoscopic abdominal surgery. Conversion was necessary in two cases due to pelvic adhesions secondary to endometriosis and inflammation, respectively.

The intra- and postoperative complication rate was reasonably low, and the consequent hospital stay was short.

10.7 Discussion and Conclusions

In cases requiring emergency surgery the laparoscopic approach for gynecologic conditions has the advantage over laparotomy of a shorter hospitalization and a faster recovery. Moreover, laparoscopy enables a comprehensive and thorough exploration of the entire abdominal cavity to confirm the preoperative diagnostic hypothesis. The laparoscopic approach also allows the treatment of different diseases by using the same surgical access, reducing the risk of post-surgical adhesions and wound complications. Laparoscopy does not affect the clinical outcome or increase the risk of impaired treatment of misdiagnosed malignant disease, requiring a second surgery [31].

In a pregnant woman laparoscopy and laparotomy may increase the possibility of spontaneous abortion in the first trimester and premature delivery in the last trimester of pregnancyrespectively. It is however common opinion that the use of laparoscopy is preferable to laparotomy. In this regard the advantages of laparoscopy over open surgery are represented by a reduced administration of anesthetic drugs, a reduced need for postoperative analgesia, a low incidence of infective complications and a faster recovery. Major risks of surgery in pregnant women include uterine injuries due to the increased uterine size, with or without rupture of the amniotic membrane, bleeding and gaseous embolism, as well as technical difficulties related to the limited working space [32, 33].

Therefore, when operating on a pregnant woman, all the necessary precautions must be taken prior to the use of laparoscopy including a low intra-abdominal pressure and deep vein thrombosis prophylactic measures even for minor procedures.

As mentioned above, when suspecting a pregnancy, handing of the uterine cavity should be completely avoided.

In the event of the incidental finding of a gynecologic disease, consultation with an experienced gynecologist is advisable. If a malignancy is suspected, it is important to remember that an inappropriate surgical approach due to inexperience can cause tumor dissemination and worsening of prognosis.

In conclusion, it is important to remember that the multi-disciplinary approach to the patient is essential for establishing the correct diagnosis and treatment in the shortest time possible and to minimize future legal concerns. The use of modern laboratory and radiologic resources associated with the progress in endoscopic surgical techniques provide both general surgeons and gynecologists with all the means necessary to ensure the best surgical result.

References

1. Semm K (1983) Endoscopic appendectomy. Endoscopy 15:59
2. Homer MJ, Braver JM (1979) Reccurrent appendicitis: reexamination of controversial disease. Gastroent Radiol 4:295
3. Van Dalen R, Bagshaw PF, Dobbs BR et al (2003) The utility of laparoscopy in the diagnosis of acute appendicitis in women of reproductive age. Surg Endosc 17:1311-1313
4. Casciola L, Ceccarelli G, Batoli A et al (2002) Approccio laparoscopico versus laparotomia per sospetta appendicite acuta. Giorn Chir 23:440-444
5. Promecene PA (2002) laparoscopy in gynaecologic emergencies. Semin Laaprosc Surg 9:64-75
6. Lopez Rivadeneyra E, Gutierrez Garcia V et al Diagnostic and therapeutic usefulness of laparoscopic surgery in acute abdomen of gynaecologic origin. Ginecol Obstet Mex 66:377-380
7. Kontoravdis A, Chryssikopoulos A, Hassiakos D et al The diagnsotic value of laparoscopy in 2365 patients with acute and chronic pelvic pain. Int J Gynecol Obstet 52:243-248
8. Henry-Suchet J (2000) PID: clinical and laparoscopic aspects. Ann N Y Acad Sci 900:301-308
9. Porpora MG, Gomel V. The role of laparoscopy in the management of pelvic pain in women of reproductive age. Fertil Steril 1998; 70:592-3
10. Eschenbach D, Woelner-Hanssen P, Hawes SE et al (1997) Acute pelvic inflammatory disease: associations of clinical and laboratory findings with laparoscopic findings. Obstet Gynecol 89:184-192
11. Pavletic AJ, Wolner-Hanssen P, Paavonen J et al (1999) Infertility following pelvic inflammatory disease. Infect Dis Obstet Gynecol 7:145-152
12. Gogate A, Barabin L, Nicholas S et al (1998) Risk factors for laparoscopically confirmed pelvic inflammatory disease: findings from Mumbai (Bombay), India. Sex Transm Inf 74:426-432
13. Buchweitz O, Malik E, Kressin P et al (2000) Laparoscopic management of tubo-ovarian abscesses. Surg Endosc 14:948-950
14. Simms I, Warburton F, Westrom L (2003) Diagnosis of pelvic inflammatory disease: time for a rethink. Sex Transm Infect 79:491-494
15. The Royal College of Obstetrician & Gynaecologist (2003) Clinical Green Top Guidelines: Management of Acute Pelvic Inflammatory Disease. Guideline No. 32. Available at: http://www.gyninfonet.com/AGCT/PDF/Pelvic_Inflamatory_Disease_No32.pdf. Accessed on 17 June 2011
16. Sau A, Hamilton-Fairley D (2003) Review: Nonsurgical diagnosis and management of ectopic pregnancy. Obstetrician & Gynaecologist 5:29-33
17. Lau S, Tulandi T (1999) Conservative medical and surgical management of interstitial ectopic pregnancy. Fertil Steril 72:207-215
18. Lundorff P (1997) Laparoscopic surgery in ectopic pregnancy. Acta Obstet Gynecol Scand 76:81-84
19. Bateman BG (1998) Laparascopic treatment in gynecologic emergencies. In: Schirmer D, Ratner WD (eds) Ambulatory Surgery, Saunders, Philadelphia
20. ASRM Practice Guideline (1997) Classification of endometriosis. Fertil Steril 67:817-821

21. Darwish AM, Zhakhera M, Youssef AA (2007) Fertility after laparoscopic management of gynecologic emergencies: the experience of a developing country. Gynecol Surg 4:85-90
22. Mol BWJ, Hajenius PJ, Engelsbel S et al (1997) An economic evaluation of laparoscopy and open surgery in the treatment of tubal pregnancy. Acta Obstet Gynecol Scand 76:596-600
23. Pan HS, Huang LW, Lee CY et al (2004) Ovarian pregnancy torsion. Arch Gynecol Obstet 270:119-121
24. Sozen I, Kadako R, Fleischman S, Arici A (2002) Diagnosis and laparoscopic management of a fallopian tube torsion following Irving tubal sterilization: a case report. Surg Endosc 16:217
25. Cohen SB, Oelser G, Seidman DS et al (1999) Laparoscopic detorsion allow sparing of the twisted ischemic adnexa. J Am Assoc Gynecol Laparosc 6:139-143
26. Martinez-Serna T, Starter KD, Filini CJ, Tomonaga T (1998) An unusual case of endometrial trocar site implantation. Surg Endosc 12:992-994
27. Chew S, Chan C, Ng SC, Ratman SS (1998) Laparoscopic adhesiolysis for subfertility. Singapore Med J 39:491-495
28. Mettler L (2003) Pelvic adhesions: laparoscopic approach. Ann N Y Acad Sci 997:255-268
29. Piscaglia F, Vidili G, Ugolini G et al (2005) Fitz-Hugh-Curtis-syndrome mimicking acute cholecystitis: value of new ultrasound findings in the differential diagnosis. Ultrashall Med 26:227-230
30. Gandhi SG, Komenaka IK, Naim JH (2003) Fitz-Hugh-Curtis syndrome after laparoscopic tubal ligation. A case report. J Reprod Med 48:302-305
31. Parker WH (1995) The case for laparoscopic management of the adnexal mass. Clin Obstet Gynecol 38:362-369
32. Barnett MB, Liu DTY (1974) Complication of laparoscopy during early pregnancy. Br Med J 1:328
33. Yuen PM, Chang AM (1997) Laparoscopic management of adnexal mass during pregnancy. Acta Obstet Gynecol Scand 76:173-176
34. Catena F, Ceccarelli G, Sartelli M (2009) Sindromi aderenziali addominali. Alpes Editori, Roma

Suggested Readings

Sauerland S, Agresta F, Bergamaschi R, Borzellino G, Budzynski A, Champault G, Fingerhut A, Isla A, Johansson M, Lundorff P (2006) Laparoscopy for abdominal emergencies. Evidence-based guidelines of the European Association for Endoscopic Surgery. Surg Endosc 20:14–29

Agresta F, Ansaloni L, Baiocchi L, Bergamini C, Campanile FB, Carlucci M, Cocorullo G, Corradi A, Franzato B, Lupo M, Mandalà V, Mirabella A, Pernazza G, Piccoli M, Staudacher C, Vettoretto N, Zago M, Lettieri E, Levati A, Pietrini D, Scaglione M, De Masi S, De Placido G, Francucci M, Rasi M, Scaramuzza G, Del Favero AL (2011) Consensus Development Conference of the Società Italiana Chirurgia Endoscopica e nuove tecnologie (SICE); Associazione Chirurghi Ospedalieri Italiani (ACOI); Società Italiana di Chirurgia (SIC); Società Italiana Chirurgia d'Urgenza e Trauma (SICUT), Società Italiana Chirurghi dell'Ospedalità Privata (SICOP) and the European Association for Endoscopic Surgery (EAES). In press

Nonspecific Abdominal Pain 11

Mario Morino and Federico Famiglietti

11.1 Definition and Epidemiology

Nonspecific abdominal pain (NSAP) is not a defined disease, but is a collection of conditions. The term NSAP refers to an abdominal or pelvic pain of less than 7 days' duration for which the diagnosis remains uncertain after clinical examination and baseline investigations [1]. Clearly, it must not be accompanied by signs of peritonitis, hemodynamic instability, or other obvious clinical presentation requiring urgent intervention.

Although it is a diagnosis of exclusion, NSAP is a very common condition. It has been reported as one of the most common diagnoses in patients suffering from abdominal pain attending emergency departments. In this setting, it may account for up to 45% of emergency admissions [2–5] with an incidence rate that reached 182 cases per 100,000 person-year in the 1990s [6]. Its frequency however is both age and sex-related, falling to 15% in patients aged over 50 years [7] and to 25% in males with a male/female ratio of 1:3 [8]. Among young women NSAP can be caused by a great number of conditions, including pelvic inflammatory disease (PID), appendicitis, ectopic pregnancy, torsion of the ovary, and endometriosis. Reaching a diagnosis is particularly challenging in these patients because of the physiologic changes associated with ovulation and menstruation that can cover symptoms of more serious conditions. In fact, the chance of missing the diagnosis might be as high as 45% in women of childbearing age.

Given this low diagnostic accuracy, many patients will be discharged from hospital after a stay of 4-6 days still without a clear diagnosis. Moreover, the length of stay could be even longer for patients aged over 70 years who also

M. Morino (✉)
Digestive and Colorectal Surgery, Centre for Minimally Invasive Surgery, University of Turin
Turin, Italy

V. Mandalà, *The Role of Laparoscopy in Emergency Abdominal Surgery*,

undergo multiple investigations more frequently than younger patients [5]. It is therefore necessary to reduce the admission rate for NSAP because of the costs and morbidity associated with this condition in terms of excessive hospital stay, multiple investigations and unnecessary surgical explorations [8, 9]. Computer-aided diagnostic questionnaires [10], abdominal ultrasound (US) [11], abdominal computed tomography (CT) [12] and early laparoscopy (EL) [13–17] have all been described as potential methods for improving the diagnostic accuracy in the emergency setting.

Nevertheless, the most important part of the evaluation remains a thorough history and a careful physical examination given the wide variety of disorders which may cause abdominal pain. The physician is called to establish a differential diagnosis, plan appropriate imaging studies and determine whether surgery is necessary.

As stated by Poulin et al., the *management of acute NSAP needs to be periodically adjusted to get the best outcomes at the lowest costs and with the least invasive and most appropriate diagnostic tools* [18]. Briefly, the management of acute NSAP can be divided into 3 stages. The first stage is the initial history, physical examination, baseline investigations, and formulation of a working and differential diagnosis. The second stage involves the judicious use of radiologic techniques. The third stage should be represented by diagnostic laparoscopy.

11.2 Baseline Investigations

Baseline bedside evaluation is essential for formulating an accurate differential diagnosis and proper preoperative workup. A detailed history should be obtained. The onset, character, intensity, location, duration and chronology of pain must be carefully evaluated. Special attention should be given to young females with right lower quadrant pain, as misdiagnosis predominantly occurs in this kind of patient. In fact, as appendicitis is the second most common diagnosis in patients with acute abdominal pain, misdiagnoses in women of reproductive age result in high rates of negative appendectomies, with longer hospital stays and more complications when compared with patients with appendicitis [19] (Figs. 11.1-11.3).

A complete blood count with differential is useful to exclude leukocytosis. Other helpful laboratory studies include: measurement of serum electrolytes, blood urea, amylase and bilirubin, urinalysis, pregnancy test and abdominal radiograph. US should be included among the baseline investigations as it has become a valuable primary imaging tool in the assessment of acute pelvic pain in women both for gynecologic and non-gynecologic diseases [20, 21]. Use of this inexpensive and fast diagnostic tool as an extension of the physical examination allows the surgeon to receive immediate information about the patient's disease process and thus permits expedited patient management. Furthermore, US does not involve radiation and is superior to CT in the evaluation of the female reproductive system.

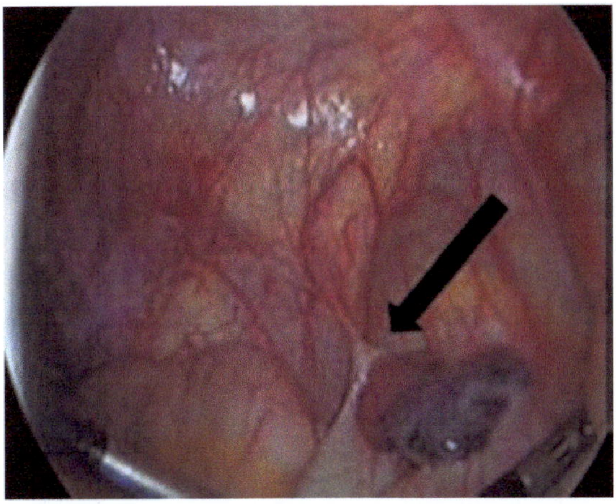

Fig. 11.1 A 42-year-old female patient. Recurrent abdominal pain in right iliac fossa for two years. Fever during the last episode. Diagnostic laparoscopy: Twists with venous stasis of epiploic appendix and infarction. Observation V. Mandalà

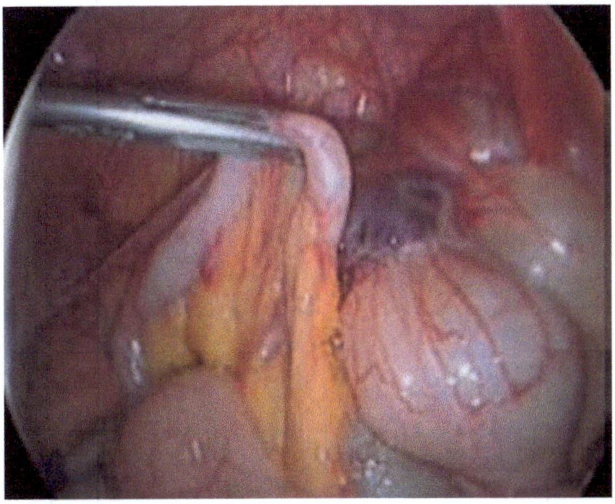

Fig. 11.2 Normal cecal appendix

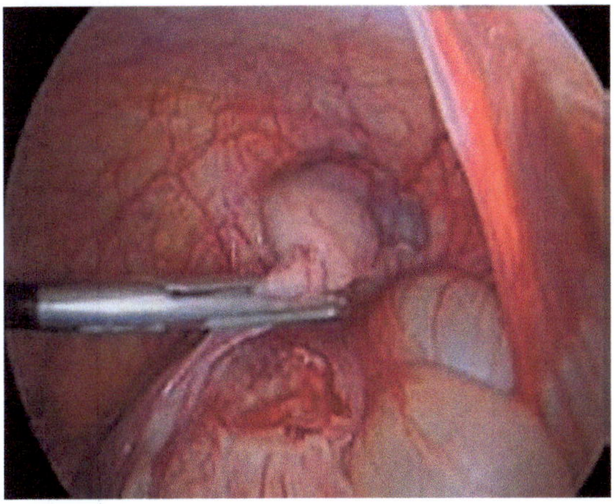

Fig. 11.3 Therapeutic laparoscopy: dissection of epiploic appendix and resection of the base

Table 11.1 Criteria adopted for specific diagnoses excluding NSAP. From [16]

Diagnoses	Criteria
Acute appendicitis	Pain and positive Blumberg sign in right lower quadrant, T >38°C, WBC >10,000 cell/mm^3
Inflammatory bowel disease	Previous diagnosis or US evidence
Ectopic pregnancy	US evidence or positive pregnancy test
Salpingitis	US evidence of collection or salpingeal empyema with clinical evidence
Endometriosis	Previous diagnosis or US evidence of nonhomogeneous cysts
Urinary infection, renal colic	Blood or leukocytes at urinalysis or US or radiologic evidence of renal stones or dilatation of urinary tract
Ovarian cyst, uterine fibroma	Cyst or fibroma >5 cm at US
IUD	Presence of IUD and vaginal loss suggestive for endometritis

T, Body Temperature; *WBC*, White Blood Cells; *US*, Ultrasound; *IUD*, Intrauterine Device.

The presence of fever, leukocytosis (WBC>10,000 cell/mm^3), or clinical signs of peritonitis, hemodynamic instability, or other obvious clinical presentation requiring urgent intervention rules out NSAP. Again, NSAP should be excluded when a specific diagnosis of right lower quadrant pain is made (Table 11.1). If at this stage a diagnosis is not made, high-quality imaging studies should be used.

11.3 Imaging Studies

Until recently, radiologic evaluation of acute abdominal pain included plain films of the abdomen and chest radiographs as the only aids for an admitting emergency physician. Nowadays more accurate technologies are available. Nevertheless, an understanding of the limitations of different radiologic techniques is needed, so that their use is appropriate and cost-effective, and avoids multiple procedures. There are situations in which the abdominal radiograph continues to play a role, for example, in detecting pneumoperitoneum or identifying small bowel obstruction. Further studies in these situations are not always required and a surgical exploration can be performed early. However, when the diagnosis remains uncertain, without the benefit of diagnostic aids such as CT scans and US, the rate of unnecessary laparotomies is often unacceptably high. For this reason in many centers CT scan has become the primary imaging technique for the evaluation of the patient with acute abdominal pain and a confused clinical picture [12, 22, 23]. It has been reported as the single best predictor of the need for urgent intervention [22]. History and clinical examination with the addition of laboratory tests and abdominal radiographs do not reach a sufficient level of sensitivity and specificity to lead to a proper management of NSAP (56% and 81%, respectively) [8, 22]. An early use of CT in the diagnostic workup of acute abdominal pain has led to a correct diagnosis in 96.8% of cases [23]. Despite concerns about its costs, it has been reported also as cost-effective by reducing the hospital stay and preventing unnecessary appendectomy [12]. However there are certain settings in which US should be preferred. When a gallstone disease is suspected, US provides more accurate information than CT (i.e. the presence of gallstones or common bile duct stones and the bile duct size). Moreover in certain patients such as children or pregnant women, US should be considered the method of choice because of concerns about radiation dose. Current guidelines for CT and MRI use during pregnancy state that pelvic CT studies should be avoided in all trimesters of pregnancy unless absolutely necessary, because of the childhood cancer risk. However, if US proves inconclusive, a CT should be considered to guide treatment and avoid harmful delays [21, 24]. Another limitation of this technique is its limited availability at all times in an emergency setting. Therefore, if the diagnosis is still uncertain or CT is not accessible, the next stage of the management of NSAP should be EL.

11.4 Early Laparoscopy versus Active Observation

An admitting emergency clinician should roughly categorize patients affected by NSAP into three groups according to findings from baseline investigations and imaging studies: patients requiring an operation, patients that can be managed conservatively and lastly patients in whom the need for surgery remains uncertain. In the latter group the severity of symptoms determines the need for emergency surgery. If symptoms are severe enough to require surgical exploration, this should be done laparoscopically [25]. The main intraoperative findings at EL are listed in Table 11.2.

However, it should be kept in mind that only a minority of all patients affected by abdominal pain will require emergency surgery and the surgical decision making is not as straightforward as it may appear. To operate on patients whose diagnosis is still doubtful can lead to a high rate of negative

Table 11.2 Intraoperative diagnosis at early laparoscopy. Modified from [16]

Diagnosis	Percentage (%)
Acute appendicitis	30.2
No diagnosis	20.7
Ovarian cyst	18.9
PID + salpingitis	15.1
Adhesions	7.5
Ectopic pregnancy	1.8
Endometriosis	1.8
Carcinoid tumor	1.8

PID, Pelvic Inflammatory Disease.

findings on surgical exploration. On the other hand, a wait-and-see policy could lead to delays in treatment resulting in high morbidity and complication rates. Owing to its high diagnostic accuracy and low morbidity and mortality compared to open surgery, EL can play a major role in establishing the correct diagnosis and reducing the need for laparotomies in this setting.

Whether EL or active observation should be preferred in patients with NSAP is largely debated in the literature. Apart from retrospective or prospective case series [26–32], the role of EL in patients with NSAP has been investigated in several randomized controlled studies (RCTs) [13–17], two meta-analyses [33, 34] and a further two systematic reviews [35, 36]. Table 11.3 gives the main outcomes of the RCTs. EL has a diagnostic accuracy that ranges from 79.2% to 96.9 with a therapeutic role up to 86.5% of cases, with low rates of morbidity (0–23.7%) and mortality (0–1.6%) when compared to those reported with laparotomy in an emergency situation. Analysis of the available data clearly showed that EL has several advantages over active observation [34]. EL has a higher rate of specific diagnosis before discharge associated with shorter hospital stay. EL was also found to be cost-effective, as if a diagnosis could be made early, there would be a large saving in resources. An improvement of quality of life in the EL group was also seen.

Despite these benefits, it should be underlined that up to 51% of patients undergoing conservative management will be operated on during the same admission or during the follow up. These patients can be safely managed laparoscopically, with a very low morbidity [16]. Therefore, delaying surgery in NSAP patients does not increase operative risks or jeopardize clinical results. Furthermore, it was reported that 49% of patients managed conservatively avoided a surgical procedure under general anesthesia without increased morbidity [16, 33, 34]. Nevertheless, the great diagnostic accuracy of EL does not show clear clinical benefits, and does not lead to a significant reduction in symptoms recurrence at long-term follow-up [15, 16].

11.5 Conclusions

In conclusion, selective indication to laparoscopy after a short period of active observation (24 to 72 hours) reduces the need for surgery without significant clinical disadvantages in patients affected by NSAP. Open surgery has a very limited role in the management of NSAP, as it is associated with low diagnostic accuracy, high morbidity and costs, and long hospital stay. Our opinion is in close agreement with the EAES guidelines on the management of NSAP, which state: *It seems justified to lower the threshold for surgical exploration when using a laparoscopic rather than an open approach. However, it seems advisable to observe patients over some hours because abdominal symptoms may become more specific over time or simply disappear in some cases* [25].

Nevertheless, in this context it is indispensable to highlight that although there have been advances in imaging techniques and laparoscopic expertise

Table 11.3 Main outcomes from RCTs. Modified from [36]

Study	Group	N.	Diagnostic accuracy (%)	Therapeutic procedures (%)	No diagnosis (%)	Persisting NSAP (%)	Morbidity (%) NSA	Mortality (%)	Mean hospital stay (days)
Champault	EL	33	96.9	63.6	3.0	-	0		4.18
1993	OBS	32	28.1	15.6	71.8		-	-	6.6
Decadt	EL	59	81.3	64.5	18.6	28.8	23.7	1.6	2
1999	OBS	61	36.0	72.7	63.9	32.7	31.1	1.6	2
Gaitan	EL	55	81.7	10.9	18.1	-	10.9	0	1.3
2002	OBS	55	8.1	12.7	21.8		9	0	2.3
Morino	EL	53	79.2	33.9	20.7	13.2	3.7	0	3.7
2006	OBS	51	45.0	7.8	54.9	47.0	1.9	0	4.7
Schietroma	EL	260	95.6	86.5	4.2	-	1.1	0	1.7
2007	OBS	262	65.2	41.2	34.7		27	0.38	7.3

EL, Early Laparoscopy; *OBS*, Active Clinical Observation; *N*, Number of patients; *NSAP*, Nonspecific Abdominal Pain.

over the years, a substantial proportion of patients ranging from 3% to 20.7% is still discharged without a specific diagnosis, and up to 28.8% of patients could experience persisting NSAP, even when EL is performed [14–17]. Outpatient evaluation with an adequate scheduled follow-up may be an option in this subgroup of patients, as it has not been associated with an increased incidence of complications and dissatisfaction [37].

References

1. de Dombal FT, Leaper DJ, Staniland JR et al (1972) Computer-aided diagnosis of acute abdominal pain. Br Med J 2:9-13
2. Brewer BJ, Golden GT, Hitch DC et al (1976) Abdominal pain. An analysis of 1,000 consecutive cases in a University Hospital emergency room. Am J Surg 131:219-223
3. Wilson DH, Wilson PD, Walmsley RG et al (1977) Diagnosis of acute abdominal pain in the accident and emergency department. Br J Surg 64:250-254
4. de Dombal FT (1986) The OMGE acute abdominal pain survey. Progress report. Scand J Gastroenterol 144:35-42
5. Irvin TT (1989) Abdominal pain: a surgical audit of 1190 emergency admissions. Br J Surg 76:1121-1125
6. Campbell WB, Lee EJ, Van de Sijpe K et al (2002) A 25-year study of emergency surgical admissions. Ann R Coll Surg Engl 84:273-277
7. Telfer S, Fenyö G, Holt PR et al (1988) Acute abdominal pain in patients over 50 years of age. Scand J Gastroenterol Suppl 144:47-50
8. Sheridan WG, White AT, Havard T et al (1992) Non-specific abdominal pain: the resource implications. Ann R Coll Surg Engl 74:181-185
9. Raheja SK, McDonald PJ, Taylor I (1990) Non-specific abdominal pain—an expensive mystery. J R Soc Med 83:10-11
10. Adams ID, Chan M, Clifford PC et al (1986) Computer aided diagnosis of acute abdominal pain: a multicentre study. BMJ 293:800-804
11. Allemann F, Cassina P, Röthlin M et al (1999) Ultrasound scans done by surgeons for patients with acute abdominal pain: a prospective study. Eur J Surg 165:966-970
12. Rao PM, Rhea JT, Novelline RA et al (1998) Effect of computed tomography of the appendix on treatment of patients and use of hospital resources. N Engl J Med 338:141-146
13. Champault G, Rizk N, Lauroy J et al (1993) Right iliac fossa pain in women. Conventional diagnostic approach versus primary laparoscopy. A controlled study (65 cases). Ann Chir 47:316-319
14. Decadt B, Sussman L, Lewis MP et al (1999) Randomized clinical trial of early laparoscopy in the management of acute non-specific abdominal pain. Br J Surg 86:1383-1386
15. Gaitán H, Angel E, Sánchez J et al (2002) Laparoscopic diagnosis of acute lower abdominal pain in women of reproductive age. Int J Gynaecol Obstet 76:149-158
16. Morino M, Pellegrino L, Castagna E et al (2006) Acute nonspecific abdominal pain: A randomized, controlled trial comparing early laparoscopy versus clinical observation. Ann Surg 244:881-886
17. Schietroma M, Carlei F, Cappelli S et al (2007) "Acute abdomen": early laparoscopy or active laparotomic-laparoscopic observation- Hepatogastroenterology 54:1137-1141
18. Poulin EC, Schlachta CM, Mamazza J (2000) Early laparoscopy to help diagnose acute nonspecific abdominal pain. Lancet 355:861-863
19. Flum DR, Koepsell T (2002) The clinical and economic correlates of misdiagnosed appendicitis: nationwide analysis. Arch Surg 137:799-804
20. Bau A, Atri M (2000) Acute female pelvic pain: ultrasound evaluation. Semin Ultrasound CT MR 21:78-93

21. Butala P, Greenstein AJ, Sur MD et al (2010) Surgical management of acute right lower-quadrant pain in pregnancy: a prospective cohort study. J Am Coll Surg 211:490-494
22. Gerhardt RT, Nelson BK, Keenan S et al (2005) Derivation of a clinical guideline for the assessment of nonspecific abdominal pain: the Guideline for Abdominal Pain in the ED Setting (GAPEDS) Phase 1 Study. Am J Emerg Med 23:709-717
23. Strömberg C, Johansson G, Adolfsson A (2007) Acute abdominal pain: diagnostic impact of immediate CT scanning. World J Surg 31:2347-2354
24. Chen MM, Coakley FV, Kaimal A et al (2008) Guidelines for computed tomography and magnetic resonance imaging use during pregnancy and lactation. Obstet Gynecol 112:333-340
25. Sauerland S, Agresta F, Bergamaschi R et al (2006) Laparoscopy for abdominal emergencies: evidence-based guidelines of the European Association for Endoscopic Surgery. Surg Endosc 20:14-29
26. Sugarbaker PH, Sanders JH, Bloom BS et al (1975) Preoperative laparoscopy in diagnosis of acute abdominal pain. Lancet 1:442-445
27. Vander Velpen GC, Shimi SM, Cuschieri A (1994) Diagnostic yield and management benefit of laparoscopy: a prospective audit. Gut 35:1617-1621
28. Cuesta MA, Eijsbouts QA, Gordijn RV et al (1998) Diagnostic laparoscopy in patients with an acute abdomen of uncertain etiology. Surg Endosc 12:915-917
29. Kirshtein B, Roy-Shapira A, Lantsberg L et al (2003) The use of laparoscopy in abdominal emergencies. Surg Endosc 17:1118-1124
30. Golash V, Willson PD (2005) Early laparoscopy as a routine procedure in the management of acute abdominal pain: a review of 1,320 patients. Surg Endosc 19:882-885
31. Agresta F, Mazzarolo G, Ciardo LF et al (2008) The laparoscopic approach in abdominal emergencies: has the attitude changed- : A single-center review of a 15-year experience. Surg Endosc 22:1255-1262
32. Karamanakos SN, Sdralis E, Panagiotopoulos S et al (2010) Laparoscopy in the emergency setting: a retrospective review of 540 patients with acute abdominal pain. Surg Laparosc Endosc Percutan Tech 20:119-124
33. Maggio AQ, Reece-Smith AM, Tang TY et al (2008) Early laparoscopy versus active observation in acute abdominal pain: systematic review and meta-analysis. Int J Surg 6:400-403
34. Gaitán HG, Reveiz L, Farquhar C (2011) Laparoscopy for the management of acute lower abdominal pain in women of childbearing age. Cochrane Database Syst Rev 1:CD007683
35. Stefanidis D, Richardson WS, Chang L et al (2009) The role of diagnostic laparoscopy for acute abdominal conditions: an evidence-based review. Surg Endosc 23:16-23
36. Domínguez LC, Sanabria A, Vega V et al (2011) Early laparoscopy for the evaluation of nonspecific abdominal pain: a critical appraisal of the evidence. Surg Endosc 25:10-8
37. Onur OE, Guneysel O, Unluer EE et al (2008) "Outpatient follow-up" or "Active clinical observation" in patients with nonspecific abdominal pain in the Emergency Department. A randomized clinical trial. Minerva Chir 63:9-15

Suggested Readings

Sauerland S, Agresta F, Bergamaschi R, Borzellino G, Budzynski A, Champault G, Fingerhut A, Isla A, Johansson M, Lundorff P (2006) Laparoscopy for abdominal emergencies. Evidence-based guidelines of the European Association for Endoscopic Surgery. Surg Endosc 20:14–29

Agresta F, Ansaloni L, Baiocchi L, Bergamini C, Campanile FB, Carlucci M, Cocorullo G, Corradi A, Franzato B, Lupo M, Mandalà V, Mirabella A, Pernazza G, Piccoli M, Staudacher C, Vettoretto N, Zago M, Lettieri E, Levati A, Pietrini D, Scaglione M, De Masi S, De Placido G, Francucci M, Rasi M, Scaramuzza G, Del Favero AL (2011) Consensus Development Conference of the Società Italiana Chirurgia Endoscopica e nuove tecnologie (SICE); Associazione Chirurghi Ospedalieri Italiani (ACOI); Società Italiana di Chirurgia (SIC); Società Italiana Chirurgia d'Urgenza e Trauma (SICUT), Società Italiana Chirurghi dell'Ospedalità Privata (SICOP) and the European Association for Endoscopic Surgery (EAES). In press

Intestinal Bleeding and Laparoscopy

12

Annunziato Tricarico, Gabriele Salvatore, Gianluca Lanni,
Raffaele Landi and Vincenzo Mandalà

12.1 Introduction

Digestive hemorrhage constitutes a broad chapter in urgent surgical disease, with a high incidence of hospital admission, about 1–3% [1] in some series, and a mortality rate of 10%. Bleeding lesions are various, as well as their sites, signs and initial symptoms. Regarding sites, hemorrhages can originate at any point along the digestive tract. Nonetheless, a classification in *upper* bleedings (i.e. proximal to the ligament of Treitz) and *lower* bleedings (i.e. distal to the ligament of Treitz) is justified by the different kind of presentation and incidence of the disease. Upper gastrointestinal bleeding (UGIB) has a global incidence [2] of 80% and the typical signs are hematemesis and/or melena; the most frequent diseases responsible for UGIB include:

- esophageal varices (25%);
- peptic ulcer (45%);
- hemorrhagic gastritis (20%);
- mallory Weiss syndrome (5%).

The remaining 5% of UGIB are defined rare [3] and include:

- gastric cancer;
- esophagitis;
- esophageal and/or duodenal diverticula;
- hiatus hernia;
- aortoduodenal fistula;
- dieulafoy syndrome;
- anastomotic ulcer;
- anticoagulant treatment.

A. Tricarico (✉)
Head of General Surgery and Laparoscopic Unit, "San Giuliano" Hospital, ASL Na2 Nord, Giugliano (NA), Italy

Lower gastrointestinal bleeding (LGIB) has a global incidence of 20%. The typical sign is the emission of more or less digested blood right up to a clear rectorrhagia. The most frequent causes are:

- Diverticulosis (30%);
- Colorectal cancer (30%);
- Angiodysplasia (20%);
- Inflammatory bowel disease (IBD) (10% of cases).

Less frequent causes are:

- Small bowel tumors;
- Meckel diverticulum;
- Intestinal invagination;
- Volvulus;
- Colitis (ischemic, actinic, infective);
- Zollinger-Ellison syndrome;
- Metastatic localizations.

Some digestive hemorrhages originate from the ligament of Treitz up to the ileocecal valve. In agreement with many authors, we recognize these lesions and classify them as *intermediate digestive hemorrhages.*

Gastric and colonic diseases are discussed in other chapters, so in this chapter we shall concentrate on intermediate digestive hemorrhages [2, 4].

12.2 Symptoms

The clinical presentation of digestive hemorrhages is strictly related to the rapidity of blood loss, and can be classified according to two patterns: (a) anemia and acute hypovolemia pattern, whereby treating the hemodynamic imbalance is mandatory; and (b) chronic anemia pattern (Table 12.1).

Typical clinical signs in digestive hemorrhages are hematemesis [2], characterized by bright red blood if coming from the esophagus or stomach without stasis, or a dark coffee-like sediment resulting from a long stay in the stomach; melena, with the emission of a more or less fluid black stool as a

Table 12.1 Digestive bleeding classification

Massive digestive bleeding (>1500 mL in few hours)
Hematocrit level <20%; Hb <10g/dL
Shock
Need for blood transfusion: 300 mL/h up to 6 hours to support hemodynamic changes
Severe digestive bleeding (up to 1000 mL)
Hematocrit level >20 – 29%; Hb 10 g/dL
Syncopal crisis may occur
Medium digestive bleeding
Hematocrit level 30%; Hb >10 g/dL

result of blood flowing rapidly into the gastrointestinal tract; rectorrhagia with the emission of bright red and/or dark blood through the rectum. There are also some clinical cases with the presence of both hematemesis and melena which are correlated with severe hemorrhage.

12.3 Diagnosis

Identifying the source of bleeding is still a challenge for surgeons [1]. Indeed, 15% of all patients with digestive bleeding fail to show a clear hemorrhagic source and 40% of all patients with lower gastrointestinal bleeding presents more than a single hemorrhagic source [1, 5]. Effectively in the last few years technology and the development of new methods have contributed to the number of patients referred to surgery without a clear definition of the disease to be treated [6].

Diagnostic imaging is a fundamental moment in the management of digestive bleeding and it is based on:

- Endoscopy;
- Conventional radiology;
- Angiography;
- Radionuclide scanning;
- Capsule endoscopy.

12.3.1 Endoscopy

Endoscopy has a high grade of specificity [7] in the identification of upper and lower digestive lesions (74–97%) but it does not seem to be reliable in the identification of an intermediate hemorrhagic lesion. Good results have been obtained in evaluating the small bowel as far as 60 cm beyond the ligament of Treitz or; by accessing the gastrointestinal tract from the anus, it is possible to examine the small bowel as far as 200 cm from the anal verge [8, 9]. At any rate, whether a simple enteroscope or double balloon enteroscope is used, the technique does have several limitations: strong sedation is required; the operator needs to have undergone specific training; when starting from the anal verge mechanical bowel preparation is required; the distal ileum can be entered in only 30% of cases as the instrument is not rigid like a traditional colonoscope [10]; there is a significant rate of iatrogenic perforations and bleedings (about 4%); and lastly, most of the small bowel remains unexplored [11].

12.3.2 Conventional Radiology

Small bowel enema is burdened by a relatively high number of false-negative results (especially regarding superficial mucosal lesions), so the specificity of the technique is low (as low as 20%). Moreover, the impossibility of performing the enema in patients affected by serious disease has confined this technique to a second choice diagnostic option [11].

12.3.3 Helical Computed Tomography (CT)

The technique has raised new hopes in detecting the sites and nature of hemorrhagic lesions. The possibility of applying imaging subtraction techniques allows the radiologist to detect the lesions, in particular neoplastic masses. Its sensitivity in detecting intermediate bleedings [4, 5, 10, 12] is 60%. CT is also able to perform virtual ileoscopy by means of special imaging reconstruction software.

12.3.4 Selective Angiography

Selective angiography is widely performed today not only as a diagnostic technique, but also for therapeutic purposes. Angiography allows the radiologist to inject drugs or special devices able to stop the blood flow through the arteries. This method is limited because it may be useful only in patients with a bleeding greater than 0.5 mL per minute. Its specificity [12] is 47%; moreover it can only be performed in hemodynamically stable patients, while anticoagulant or antiaggregant treatment is a contraindication.

12.3.5 Radionuclide Scanning

Radioactive isotopes may be used to identify intermediate digestive bleedings with a specificity ranging from 20 to 40%. Scanning is performed with Tc_{99} mC when the hemorrhage is greater than 0.1–0.4 mL per minute [1, 9].

12.3.6 Capsule Endoscopy

Initially considered the answer to all diagnostic problems, capsule endoscopy [8, 13] has lately shown several limitations, such as the need to change batteries, the variability of intestinal peristalsis which can cause the capsule to float (sometimes too quickly), the possibility of acquiring only two frames per second and lastly the inability to track the precise location of the device within the small bowel. At any rate, this technique seems to be an important technological innovation, with a sensitivity ranging from 75 to 90%, especially in patients with intestinal bleeding of unknown etiology [7].

12.4 Laparoscopy

Of all the diagnostic techniques at the surgeon's disposal, laparoscopy plays a very important role. It can be considered at the same time the last diagnostic deed and the first therapeutic act.

When all described diagnostic techniques fail, the direct mini-invasive approach can detect the site and nature of the hemorrhage with good specificity. In fact, laparoscopic exploration of the abdominal cavity can show every morphological alteration regarding the serosal surface of the bowel, small bowel mesentery, and possible hematocele that are the expression of malformations or proliferative disease. Furthermore, taking advantage of peri-laparoscopic US scan [14], it is possible to diagnose the presence of extremely small-size masses as well as to establish the infiltration grade and the borders of the pathologic lesions. Lastly, when necessary, it is possible to perform a simultaneous laparoscopic and endoscopic approach [15–17]: an enteroscope is advanced through an ileal breach next to a hematocele to exploit the entire length of the enteroscope to study ileum. The sensitivity of this combined technique is 95% while perforative and hemorrhagic complications are about 4% as reported in the literature.

12.4.1 Technique

Usually the patient referred to the laparoscopic procedure is in the head-down position, either for diagnostic or therapeutic procedures. We pay attention to check systems and anti-decubitus devices; in fact only by changing the position of the patient (Trendelenburg, reverse Trendelenburg position, right or left rotation) can the surgeon explore the abdominal cavity and small bowel in the search for the site and nature of an intestinal hemorrhage. We make a transverse incision under the umbilicus to establish pneumoperitoneum with a Veress needle; usually we reserve open access to patients presenting both intestinal bleeding and occlusive syndrome and to patients with previous abdominal surgery.

The first trocar is placed inferior to the umbilicus to give access to a 10 mm 30° laparoscope. Under laparoscopic guidance the second and third 5/10 mm trocars are inserted at the level of the umbilicus on the right and left midclavicular lines. We insert a fourth trocar in the right iliac fossa. Under laparoscopic control we check the entire small bowel from the ileocecal valve to the ligament of Treitz with a laparoscopic bowel clamp.

Regarding resection of the affected bowel and subsequent anastomosis, we prefer to perform this after mini-laparotomy and externalization of the bowel. A 30° laparoscope is fundamental for complete vision of the abdominal cavity together with the possibility of bowel transillumination. A high flow aspirator-irrigator is decisive for the rapid clearing of the operative field and to avoid peritoneal cavity contamination.

12.4.2 Personal Experience

Our experience of intermediate gastrointestinal bleeding treated with the laparoscopic approach involved 23 patients, of whom 20 presented bleeding of unknown origin while 3 patients had a certain diagnosis of the type and location of the disease. Table 12.2 reports all the diseases treated in our department.

Twelve patients with Meckel's diverticulum (9 males) aged from 20 to 30 years presented recurrent hemorrhages. One showed symptoms of inflammatory disease (acute diverticulitis), while another patient was diagnosed with diverticulosis during a laparoscopy for leiomyosarcomas. All the patients with hemorrhage underwent endoscopic investigation (gastroscopy and colonoscopy), selective mesenteric arteriography scintigraphy with technetium 99 and (Fig. 12.1). In two cases an intra-peritoneal resection of diverticulum was performed with an Endo GIA™ universal stapler (Tyco autosuture); in the remaining cases, a mini-laparotomy was performed for resection of the pathologic loop.

In the six cases of small bowel leiomyoma (4 males) aged 25 to 32 years, the lesion presented with repeated hemorrhage. Diagnosis was made with the laparoscopic approach after the diagnostic methods mentioned above failed. Also in these cases, during the course of the same laparoscopy, a resection of the bowel loop was performed by means of a targeted mini-laparotomy, with externalization followed by a manual T-T anastomosis.

The small bowel leiomyosarcoma involved a 40-year-old male patient in whom Meckel's diverticulum had been diagnosed by CT scan, and who presented a hemorrhage associated with abdominal subocclusive syndrome. After lysis of the adherences, the lesion was externalized by means of Pfannenstiel mini-laparotomy, and an intestinal resection was performed using a manual T-T anastomosis.

In two cases of patients with a small bowel melanoma one of these patients presented a digestive hemorrhage together with an occlusive syndrome secondary to a chronic invagination close to the neoplasia. Surgical treatment in this patient was performed using the same method described above.

The last patient, a 16-year-old girl with Peutz-Jeghers syndrome, presented subocclusive symptoms together with a digestive hemorrhage. Combined video-laparoscopy and surgery were performed through a small incision to carry out resection and anastomosis.

We also treated a gastric leiomyoma which presented with hemorrhage.

Table 12.2 Personal experience

12 Meckel diverticula
1 gastric leiomyoma
1 jejunal leiomyosarcoma
6 small bowel leiomyomas
2 small bowel melanomas
1 Peutz-Jeghers syndrome

Table 12.3 Possible causes of intermediate digestive bleeding

Possible causes
Malignancy
Crohn disease
Meckel diverticulum
Enteritis (ischemic, actinic, infective)
Gastrointestinal stromal tumor
Ileal lymphoma
Metastatic localizations
Vascular malformations
Ectopic pancreas
Peutz-Jeghers syndrome
Polyposis

12.5 Discussion

The treatment options for intestinal bleeding include consolidated techniques in which the mini-invasive approach is gaining an increasingly important role in the management of the hemorrhagic patient. In the last few years the main goal has been to lower the percentage of patients referred to surgery (about 20%) without a clear location of the hemorrhage. Today the challenge has been moved and the problem is how to treat the hemorrhagic patient who is often sorely tried and sometimes debilitated by repeated episodes of intestinal bleeding. Among the various options the role of the mini-invasive laparoscopic approach has been shown to be relevant for a number of precise indications [18–20]; it allows the surgeon to manage debilitated patients suffering from many co-morbidities. At the same time it enables a more rapid postoperative recovery, a shorter hospital stay and less severe surgical trauma than does explorative laparotomy. Table 12.3 lists possible causes of intermediate digestive hemorrhage; most of these can benefit from mini-invasive treatment.

Bleeding from a Meckel diverticulum, is not a frequent event it affects 2–4% of the population and as such is the most frequent cause of rectal bleeding [21–23]. In these patients laparoscopic treatment is the gold standard: the surgical procedure consists of the removal of the diverticulum using a linear stapler and this can be performed without a service incision, thus fostering optimal patient compliance [24] (Figs. 12.2–12.4).

The treatment of ileal neoplasms (leiomyomas, leiomyosarcomas) [21] takes advantage of mini-invasive surgery; once the site of the lesion has been identified, the resection of the ileum can be done with extra-abdominal anastomosis through a focused mini-laparotomy or by creating an intra-abdominal anastomosis with an endo-GIA.

Laparoscopic treatment is also extremely useful in the so-called *rare disease*, such as pancreatic ectopy, where all the advantages of laparoscopy are exploited either in the diagnostic phase, using image magnification to see

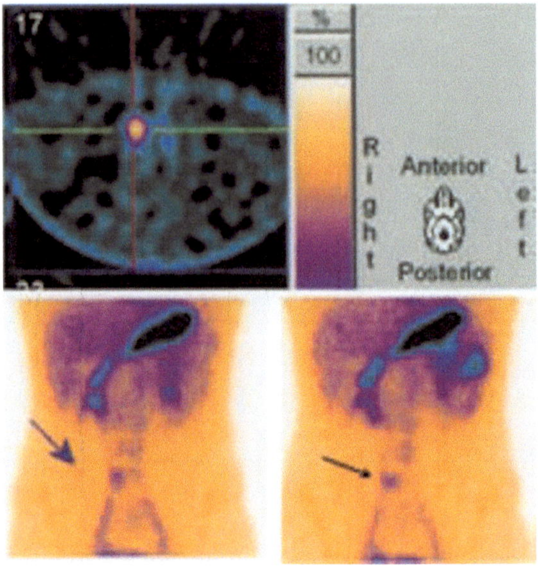

Fig. 12.1 Case report: a 16-year-old youth with previous repeated intestinal bleeding. Technetium scan: abnormal absorption in right iliac fossa. Observation V. Mandalà

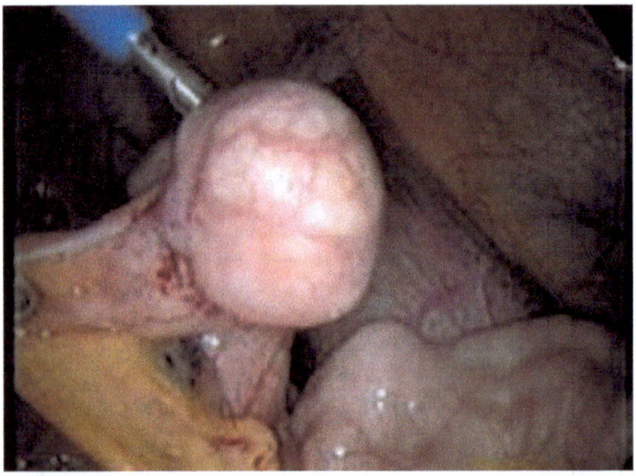

Fig. 12.2 Intraoperative laparoscopic pictures: Meckel's diverticulum with heterotopic gastric islands visible at diagnostic laparoscopy. Observation V. Mandalà

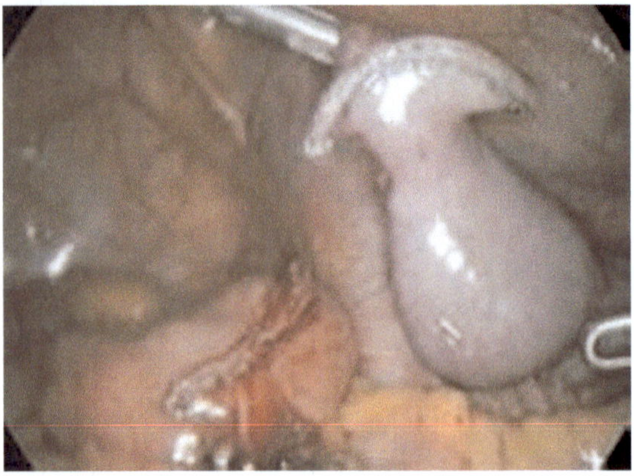

Fig. 12.3 Merckel's diverticulum removed at the base with endo-GIA

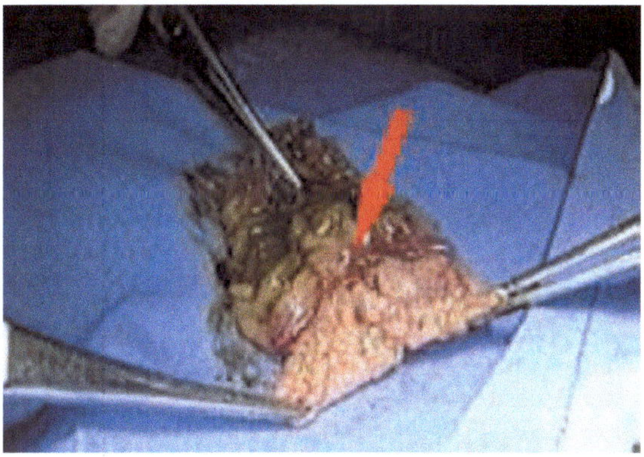

Fig. 12.4 Removal of Meckel's diverticulum by therapeutic laparoscopy. At cut surface the point of bleeding (ulcer) between the heterotopic gastric mucosa and the intestinal mucosa is visible (*arrow*). Observation V. Mandalà

ectopic islands [25], or in the treatment phase for the possibility of performing a focused ileal resection. Moreover, laparoscopy is useful in vascular malformations (angiodysplasias) [26] which can benefit, once endovascular therapy has failed, from the possibilities offered by the mini-invasive approach which span from segmental ileal resections to hemicolectomy. Lastly, bleeding in patients affected by adenomatous polyposis coli can be efficiently treated by laparoscopy as the first choice therapy. This technique allows a number of possibilities ranging from simple resections to an eventual total colectomy and ileorectal anastomosis [27], with small trauma of the gut wall and a rapid recovery from surgery.

12.6 Conclusions

Laparoscopic surgery appears to be highly useful in the management of gastrointestinal tract bleedings, particularly for those defined as *intermediate* and especially in those cases where diagnosis in uncertain, thus avoiding the need for unnecessary explorative laparotomies. Mini-invasive surgery enables the complete and thorough inspection of the bowel loops, thus contributing in combination with other methods to reaching the final diagnosis. It also enables an effective therapy combined with a small focused laparotomy. The advantages of such mini-invasive approaches have been universally acknowledged: data reported in a number of case-reports not only confirm the efficacy of the method, but they also confirm the good compliance of the patients, as shown by a shorter post-surgical hospital stay and less severe post-surgical pain.

References

1. Lee J, Costantini TW, Coimbra R (2009) Acute lower GI bleeding for the acute care surgeon: current diagnosis and management. Scand J Surg 98:135-142

2. Greer SE, Gupta R (2010) Lower gastrointestinal bleeding of unknown origin: tricks of the trade. Scand J Surg 99:103-105
3. Tricarico A, Falco P, Sozio M (2001) Emorragie digestive gravi ad eziologia rara. Rassegna dell'esperienza nazionale atti S.I.C. 1:41-52
4. Raju GS, Gerson L, Das A, Lewis B (2007) American Gastroenterological Association Institute technical review on obscure gastrointestinal bleeding. Gastroenterology 133:1697-1717
5. Czymek R, Kempf A, Roblick UJ et al (2008) Surgical treatment concepts for acute lower gastrointestinal bleeding. J Gastrointest Surg 12:2212-2220
6. Manning-Dimmitt LL, Dimmitt SG, Wilson GR (2005) Diagnosis of gastrointestinal bleeding in adults. Am Fam Physician 71:1339-1346
7. Enns R (2001) Acute lower gastrointestinal bleeding: part 1. Can J Gastroenterol 8:509-516
8. Bresci G (2009) Occult and obscure gastrointestinal bleeding: causes and diagnostic approach in 2009. World J Gastrointest Endosc 1:3-6
9. Westerof J, Weersma RK, Koornstra JJ (2009) Investigating obscure gastrointestinal bleeding: capsule endoscopy or double balloon. Neth J Med 67: 260-265
10. Saperas E (2007) Lower gastro intestinal bleeding: the great unknown. Gastroenterology Hepat 30:93-100
11. Douard R, Wind P, Panis Y et al (2000) Intraoperative enteroscopy for diagnosis and management of unexplained gastrointestinal bleeding. Am J Surg 180:181-184
12. Yamaguchi T, Yoshikawa K (2003) Enhanced CT for initial localization of active lower gastrointestinal bleeding. Abdom Imaging 28:634-636
13. Karanicolas PJ, Colquhoun PH, Dahlke E, Guyatt GH (2008) Mesenteric angiography for the localization and treatment of acute lower gastrointestinal bleeding. Can J Surg 51:437-441
14. Costamagna G, Shah SK, Riccioni ME et al (2002) A prospective trial comparing small bowel radiographs and video capsule endoscopy for suspected small bowel disease. Gastroenterology 123:999-1005
15. Novitsky YW, Kercher KW, Sing RF, Heniford BT (2006) Long-term outcomes of laparoscopic resection of gastric gastrointestinal stromal tumors. Ann Surg 243:738-747
16. Hartmann D, Schmidt H, Bolz G et al (2005) A prospective two-center study comparing wireless capsule endoscopy with intraoperative enteroscopy in patients with obscure GI bleeding. Gastrointest Endosc 61:826-832
17. Hsu PS, Chen JL, Yu JC et al (2008) Accurate diagnosis and successful treatment for massive obscure small intestinal bleeding by means of intra-operative enteroscopy: a case report. Eur J Gastroenterol Hepatol 20:139-141
18. Roldán FP, Carro PG, García MC et al (2009) Urgent intraoperative total enteroscopy with colonoscopy by means of a double enterotomy in a severe lower digestive tract haemorrhage. Cir Esp 86:252-253
19. Loh DL, Munro FD (2003) The role of laparoscopy in the management of lower gastro-intestinal bleeding. Pediatr Surg Int 19:266-267
20. Tordjman G, Bernard B, Chigot JP (1997) Recurrent lower digestive hemorrhage in young adults: a surgical indication. Gastroenterol Clin Biol 21:217-218
21. Tricarico A, Cione G, Sozio M et al (2002) Digestive hemorrhages of obscure origin. Surg Endosc 16:711-713
22. Ming-Chen Ba, San Hua Qing, Xian-Cheng Huang et al (2006) Application of laparoscopy in diagnosis and treatment of massive small intestinal bleeding: report of 22 cases. World J Gastroent 12:7051-7054
23. Fu KI, Hamahata Y, Tsujinaka Y (2010) Early colon cancer within a diverticulum treated by magnifying chromo endoscopy and laparoscopy. World J Gastroenterol 16:1545-1547
24. Bona D, Schipani LS, Nencioni M et al (2008) Laparoscopic resection for incidentally detected Meckel diverticulum. World J Gastroenterol 14:4961-4963
25. Ah-Soune P, Vitton V, Subtil C et al (2008) Ectopic pancreas: an exceptional cause of lower intestinal bleeding with hemorrhagic shock. Gastroenterol Clin Biol 32:202-204

26. Ríos A, Montoya M, Rodríguez JM, Parrilla P (2006) Severe lower gastrointestinal hemorrhage caused by colonic angiodysplasia. Diagnosis and management. Rev Esp Enferm Dig 98:625-626
27. Delgado Plasencia L, Arteaga González I, López-Tomassetti Fernández EM et al (2006) Restorative proctocolectomy with an ileoanal pouch: the role of laparoscopy. Rev Esp Enferm Ddig 98:420-428

Suggested Readings

Sauerland S, Agresta F, Bergamaschi R, Borzellino G, Budzynski A, Champault G, Fingerhut A, Isla A, Johansson M, Lundorff P (2006) Laparoscopy for abdominal emergencies. Evidence-based guidelines of the European Association for Endoscopic Surgery. Surg Endosc 20:14–29

Agresta F, Ansaloni L, Baiocchi L, Bergamini C, Campanile FB, Carlucci M, Cocorullo G, Corradi A, Franzato B, Lupo M, Mandalà V, Mirabella A, Pernazza G, Piccoli M, Staudacher C, Vettoretto N, Zago M, Lettieri E, Levati A, Pietrini D, Scaglione M, De Masi S, De Placido G, Francucci M, Rasi M, Scaramuzza G, Del Favero AL (2011) Consensus Development Conference of the Società Italiana Chirurgia Endoscopica e nuove tecnologie (SICE); Associazione Chirurghi Ospedalieri Italiani (ACOI); Società Italiana di Chirurgia (SIC); Società Italiana Chirurgia d'Urgenza e Trauma (SICUT), Società Italiana Chirurghi dell'Ospedalità Privata (SICOP) and the European Association for Endoscopic Surgery (EAES). In press

The Role of Laparoscopy in Emergency Treatment of Complications after Laparoscopic and Endoscopic Procedures

13

Francesco Corcione, Diego Cuccurullo, Felice Pirozzi, Antonio Sciuto, Camillo La Barbera and Stefano Mandalà

13.1 Introduction

Since its introduction in the late 1980s, the evolution and increasing diffusion of laparoscopic surgery has allowed the realization of a growing number of minimally invasive surgical techniques, thanks to improved technology, in terms of instruments and image transmission. Without doubt, all major abdominal surgery can be performed with a laparoscopic approach and laparoscopy is now the gold standard for surgical treatment in an increasing number of diseases [1].

13.2 State of the Art

The laparoscopic technique is not a practice without complications. Depending on the procedures performed, the incidence of reported complications ranges between 0.05% and 1.8% [2–4]. If these complications are recognized intraoperatively, they generally have a favorable course with the benefit of immediate treatment. In contrast, if the complications are detected in the postoperative course (e.g. bleeding, perforation of hollow viscera, intestinal obstruction and ischemia, infection and intra-abdominal abscess, biliary fistulas, anastomotic dehiscence), they often require – as in open surgery – a reoperation which may be associated with increased morbidity and mortality [5–7]. In these conditions, early recognition and the establishment of adequate treatment are essential factors for a favorable outcome.

F. Corcione (✉)
Department of General, Laparoscopic and Robotic Surgery,
Azienda Ospedaliera dei Colli Monaldi-Cotugno-CTO, Naples, Italy

V. Mandalà, *The Role of Laparoscopy in Emergency Abdominal Surgery*,

The main advantage of minimally invasive procedures is a shorter and smooth first operative course, with minimal pain and earlier mobilization. In this regard, it is notewarty that if the postoperative course does not follow the usual pattern , the onset of a possible complication should be suspected [5]. In such cases further investigations are needed in order to especially in the early postoperative course their confirm the existence of the suspected complication. Laboratory tests are not usually very specific and therefore their diagnostic capabilities are limited. Imaging studies are used, but findings are often non-specific and results can be misleading, negative findings do, not exclude a serious complication, while surveys with positive results (such as early detection of free air or fluid in the abdomen) are not always conclusive [3]. For example, following a laparoscopic cholecystectomy, 43% of patients have free fluid in the abdominal cavity on CT or on ultrasound, and this finding is generally devoid of pathologic significance [8].

When a postoperative complication is suspected and investigations are not conclusive, a second-look laparoscopy is advisable rather than performing an exploratory laparotomy, which could lead to greater postoperative pain and prolonged ileus and may be associated with abdominalinfections and word complications with a significant increase in length of hospital stay. In this regard, Dexter et al. [8] emphasize that a laparotomy can be avoided with a relaparoscopy in most patients with abdominal complications after laparoscopic cholecystectomy. Compared to the relaparotomy possible disadvantages of laparotomic reoperation in experienced hands is quite simple: trocar insertion can be performed through the old port situs, and if the exploration turned out to be negative, there would be no significant lengthening of postoperative recovery time. In essence, its use as a primary diagnostic modality in suspected complications can be justified.

Since laparoscopy allows a complete visualization and exploration of the abdominal cavity, it may have a role of paramount importance in recognizing the cause of the complication and treat it at the same time [2]. Even if the complication is recognized and diagnosed by non invasive examinations, the role of therapeutic laparoscopy is widely accepted, although not a large number of studies is reported in the literature [1, 9–15]. All published studies also recognize the considerable advantages that the laparoscopic approach offers compared to laparotomy and also highlight the utility of laparoscopic treatment of the complications after a recent laparotomy. In fact, avoiding relaparotomy reduces surgical trauma, resulting in a lower incidence of postoperative complications and a shorter hospital stay. An experienced team in the management of laparoscopic acute conditions is able to perform advanced laparoscopic procedures and this is the key to success in these cases [16, 17].

Some authors reach a correct diagnosis by laparoscopy in 100% of cases of postoperative complications; they also refer to have completed the operation with the minimally invasive approach in 80% of cases [2, 8, 16]. Other authors in some cases have opted for direct laparotomy reoperation in the presence of an occlusive phenomenon [18]. Overcoming the learning curve and improving techniques have enabled experienced teams to use laparoscopy in emergency conditions. In acute diseases such as ulcer perforation, colonic diverticulitis with acute complications, intestinal obstruction, as well as in emergency trauma surgery, the expert surgeon opts for the laparoscopic approach and often carries out the operation without conversion to laparotomy [9, 19–21].

The presentation of an acute abdomen is very frequent in the departments of emergency surgery and in hospitals with emergency room. A prerequisite to performing a laparoscopic approach in emergency is to have stable hemodynamic conditions: in the absence of this requirement, proceeding with an open approach is imperative [9, 19–21].

The aim is of this study to evaluate the role of laparoscopy in emergency. For this purpose we retrospectively analyze our series of minimally invasive approach in both diagnostic and therapeutic procedures in patients who had a postoperative complication or a complication after an endoscopic procedure.

13.3 Our Experience

In our clinical practice, although our hospital has no emergency room or emergency surgery, we have had to deal with acute abdominal situations in patients hospitalized in our department or in other departments. All requiring emergency treatment of post operative complications were approached laparoscopically, provided that there were no contraindications in terms of hemodynamic stability. We believe that the laparoscopic approach can be applied not only in all cases of abdominal emergencies, which have been widely described in the literature, but also for the treatment of postoperative complications.

13.3.1 Materials and Methods

From January 1999 to December 2010 a total of 9870 elective laparoscopic procedures were performed at the Department of General and Laparoscopic Surgery in Monaldi Hospital (Naples) (Table 13.1). Of these, 95 were performed with robot technology (three-arm Da Vinci Robot) and 34 with SILS and NOTES technique (transvaginal cholecystectomy). Pneumoperitoneum was established with the Tuol technique (transumbilical open laparoscopy) when umbilical access was used (cholecystectomy, appendectomy, varicocelectomy, and most cases of diagnostic laparoscopy) and open Veress-assisted techniquewas used in the remaining cases [22].

We analyzed 160 laparoscopic procedures performed in the same period for endoscopic or surgical complications. Patients included 86 women and 74 men aged between 15 and 81 years old (mean 53.7 years old).

Complications included bleeding (n=57), peritonitis (n=78) and bowel obstruction (n=25) (Table 13.2). Bleeding complications occurred in the fol-

Table 13.1 Type of primary laparoscopic surgery

Cholecystectomy and bile duct surgery	4980
Colorectal surgery	1283
TAPP	1185
Diagnostic laparoscopy	429
Surgery of the gastroesophageal junction	312
Splenectomy	300
Incisional hernia rapair	262
Gastric resection	202
Spermatic vein ligation	118
Adrenalectomy	114
Appendectomy	106
Nephrectomy	68
Distal pancreatectomy	48
Hepatectomy and liver resection	31
Esophageal resection	30
DCP	21
Others	381
Total	9870

TAPP, Transabdominal Preperitoneal Approach; *DPC*, Duodenocephalopancreasectomy.

lowing cases: 32 after cholecystectomy, seven after colorectal surgery, three after duodenocephalopancreasectomy (DPC), three after gastric resection, one after gastric resection surgery, four after splenectomy, one after nephrectomy, two after antireflux, two after transabdominal preperitoneal approach, one after ligation of the spermatic veins, and one after a diagnostic laparoscopy. Peritonitis complications occurred in the following cases: 49 after colorectal surgery, seven after cholecystectomy, two after nephrectomy, one after incisional hernia, 18 after colonoscopy and one after endoscopic retrograde cholangiopancreatography (ERCP). Bowel bostruction occurred in the following cases: 12 after colorectal surgery, three following antireflux surgery, four after incisional hernia repair, two after gastric resection, two after appedectomy and two after ileal resection.

13.3.2 Results

13.3.2.1 Bleeding

Postoperative bleeding (n=57) was managed laparoscopically in all cases. In 27 cases (47.4%) the source of active bleeding was not identified and abdominal lavage with placement of drainage tubes (mean 1.7, range 1–3) was performed. A clear improvement in the patients' clinical conditions was observed

Table 13.2 Post operative complications treated laparoscopically

Primary procedure	Complications observed		
	Bleeding (57)	Peritonitis (78)	Bowel obstruction (25)
Cholecystectomy	32	7	-
Colorectal surgery	7	49	12
Gastric resection	3	-	2
Antireflux plastic	2	-	3
Incisional hernia	-	1	4
TAPP	2	-	-
Splenectomy	4	-	-
Nephrectomy	1	2	-
DCP	3	-	-
Appendectomy	-	-	2
Ileal resection	-	-	2
Gastric bypass	1	-	-
Ligation of spermatic veins for varicocele	1	-	-
Diagnostic laparoscopy	1	-	-
Colonoscopy	-	18	-
ERCP	-	1	-

TAPP, Transabdominal Preperitoneal Approach; *DPC*, Duodenocephalopancreasectomy; *ERCP*, Endoscopic Retrograde Cholangiopancreatography.

within two hours after relaparoscopy. Fifteen patients (26.3%) had bleeding from a port site and no difference was observed between 5- and 10-mm ports. In five patients without active bleeding, the presence of clots near the trocar site suggested this was the cause of bleeding. Bleeding was controlled with bipolar coagulation in 12 cases and with suture in three cases. Seven patients (12.3%) had anastomotic bleeding, of whom three from pancreaticogastric anastomosis, probably caused by erosion of peripancreatic vessels by pancreatic secretion and four from mechanical gastrojejunal anastomosis; bleeding was managed with bipolar coagulation and/or suture.

Five patients (8.8%) had bleeding after colorectal surgery. In two cases bleeding originated from vessels of the mesocolon and it was controlled with endoloop in one case and clip placement in the other (Fig. 13.1).

One case of bleeding from the anterior surface of the pancreas was managed with bipolar coagulation and the last two cases of pelvic bleeding in the perirectal space were controlled with bipolar coagulation and/or local hemostatic agents (fibrin glue, cyanoacrylate, thrombin hemostatic matrix).

Reoperation was required in 2 cases after laparoscopic splenectomy due to bleeding from the short gastric vessels which was controlled with clip placement.

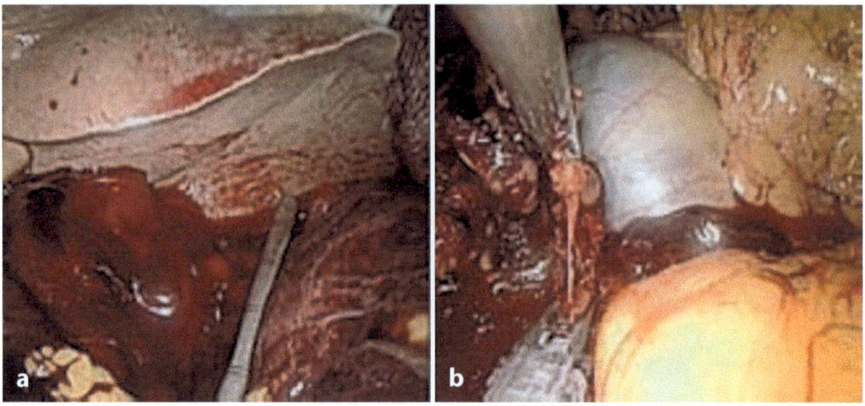

Fig. 13.1 **a** Hemoperitoneum after left hemicolectomy for bleeding from the mesocolon. **b** Clip placement on the bleeding vessel

Lastly, one case of bleeding from the greater omentum after laparoscopic cholecystectomy was managed with bipolar coagulation.

A total of 43/57 (75.4%) patients required blood transfusion before reoperation (mean 1.4 units, range 1–3) and 4/43 (9.3%) postoperatively (mean 1.1 units, range 1–2).

13.3.2.2 Peritonitis

We report 78 cases of peritonitis which were all managed laparoscopically. Forty-two patients required reoperation for anastomotic leak (Fig. 13.2) after colorectal surgery (26 after anterior resection of the rectum, nine after left hemicolectomy and seven after right hemicolectomy; the overall incidence of anastomotic leak was 3.2%). Reoperation consisted of peritoneal lavage, placement of one or more drainage tubes (mean 1.9, range 1–4), performing ileostomy (38 cases, 90.5%) or Hartmann procedure (4 cases, 9.5%).

Twenty-four patients had colonic perforation: two after laparoscopic left nephrectomy, 18 due to colonoscopy and four due to colonic ischemia after left hemicolectomy. Hartmann procedure was performed in cases of ischemic perforation. Endoscopic perforations were dealt with by direct suture repair of the defect in well-prepared bowel, early reoperation and small lesion (n=9); otherwise suture and ileostomy were performed (n=8). One case of perforation during endoscopic polypectomy was treated with resection and primary anastomosis to remove a voluminous rectosigmoid adenoma. Colonic perforation after nephrectomy was treated with lavage of the peritoneal cavity, exteriorization of the perforated colon and performance of temporary colostomy which was closed two months later.

We report two cases of jejunoileal perforation after left hemicolectomy, probably due to an erroneous traction exercised by the assistant grasp out of the field of vision. Clinical presentation was peritonitis on the 2nd postopera-

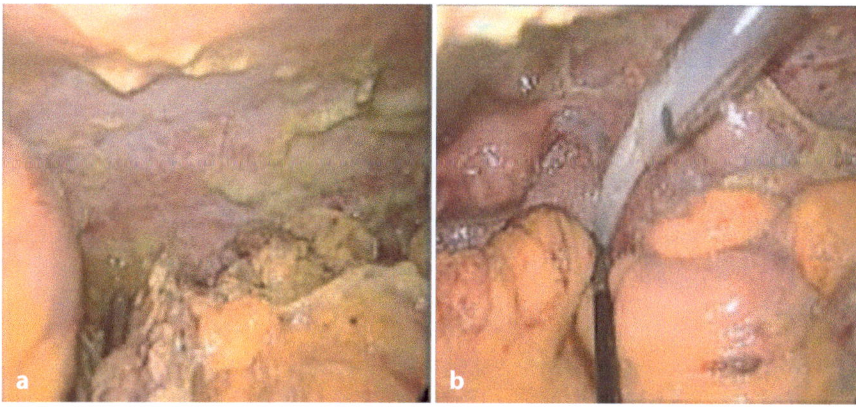

Fig. 13.2 a Peritonitis from colorectal anastomotic leak. **b** Placement of drainage tube after peritoneal lavage

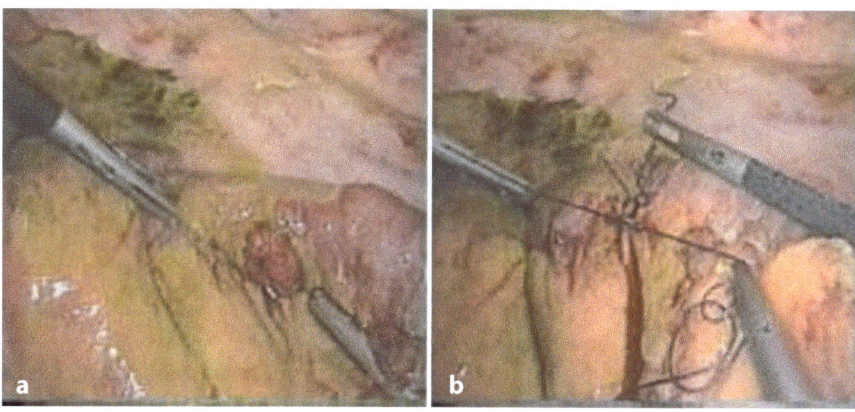

Fig. 13.3 a Peritonitis from ileal perforation during left hemicolectomy. **b** Direct repair of the defect with interrupted suture

tive day. Direct repair with interrupted suture (Fig. 13.3), abdominal lavage and drainage were performed.

We report one case of jejunal perforation after laparoscopic repair of a large incisional hernia in the right lower quadrant in an obese patient. Perforation was detected on the second postoperative day through enteric content appearing in the subcutaneous Redon drainage. We think that a delayed perforation occurred in this case, probably due to a heat injury of superficial layers of the intestinal wall with the eschar being cast off at the resumption of peristalsis. The case required abdominal lavage, direct suture repair of the defect, copious lavage of the mesh (which was ultralight and macroporous) and drainage tube placement. The postoperative course was favorable and the patient was discharged on the sixth postoperative day. Neither mesh infection nor recurrence of hernia was observed after two-years follow-up.

One case of unrecognized left ureteral partial transection during left hemicolectomy was treated with explorative laparoscopy, lavage and drainage of the abdominal cavity and stent placement.

We report seven cases of choleperitoneum after laparoscopic cholecystectomy. Two cases of bile leak from an accessory duct of the gallbladder fossa; the duct was closed with 4-0 suture and a drainage tube was placed. In four cases the source of the bile leak was not found: one required only lavage of the abdominal cavity while papillosphincterotomy was performed in 3 cases; in the last case an accessory duct injury of the 4th segment was found and managed with papillosphincterotomy and biliary stent placement.

Eleven patients had duodenal perforation after ERCP. Only the first case was managed laparoscopically. It had an unfavorable course which led to patient death on the 16th postoperative day because of sepsis. The second case was approached laparoscopically, but it required conversion because of technical difficulties. These cases led us to belive this complication should be treated early with an open approach because of the major distension of the bowel loops and the impossibility of adequate duodenal mobilization. Therefore, only one case was treated laparoscopically, while in all the others we performed laparotomy, and after duodenal mobilization, blue dye was injected through the nasogastric tube. In the four cases where a perforation was detected, it was repaired with direct suture and omentopexy, cholecystectomy was performed and a T-tube was placed. In the remaining six cases, where perforation was not evident, only drainage was placed.

13.3.2.3 Bowel Obstructions

We report 25 cases of bowel obstruction all managed laparoscopically except one. Early postoperative adhesions were the most frequent cause accounting for 14 cases: two cases of obstruction were caused by adhesions between the mesh and intestinal loops after incisional hernia repair, while the other 12 cases were due to adhesion bands (six after colorectal surgery, two after appendectomy, one after gastric resection, two after ileal resection and one after incisional hernia repair). Laparoscopic adhesiolysis was only performed in 13 cases (Fig. 13.4). One case required the resection of an ileal loop due to ischemia.

Seven cases of postoperative obstruction secondary to internal hernia were treated. In one of these cases the cause of the occlusion was the incarceration of a jejunal loop in the slit of the prosthesis after incisional hernia repair. The procedure involved the laparoscopic exploration and reduction of the incarcerated loop with careful maneuvers of traction, with no evidence of vascular damage and rapid resumption of peristalsis. The remaining six cases of occlusion due to internal hernia occurred after colorectal surgery. In one case several bowel loops had shifted below the preanastomic colic loop; since then we usually fix it to the posterior plane with fibrin glue or sutures. In three cases obstruction was caused by the incarceration of the loops in the pelvis after a

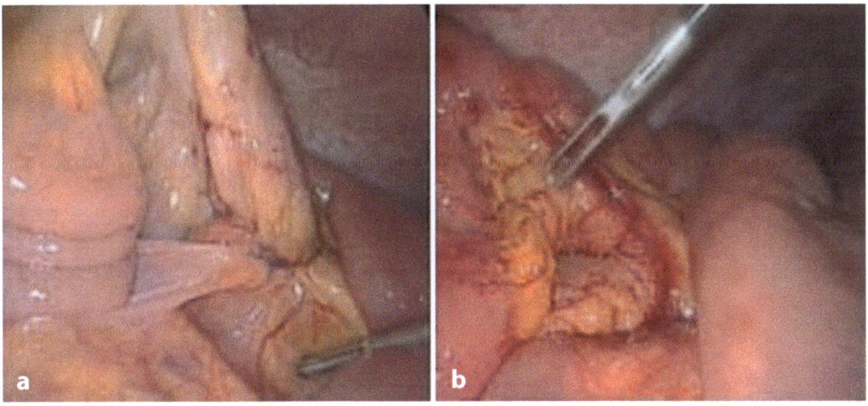

Fig. 13.4 a Obstruction due to adhesion band. **b** Adhesiolysis and release of the ileal loop

Miles abdominoperineal resection and in two cases there was lateral pinching of the bowel loops in the pelvis after anterior resection of the rectum. In six of the previous cases releasing the bowel loops was enough with resumption of vascular supply and peristalsis, whereas in one case a segmental ileal resection with direct anastomosis was required due to vascular impairment.

We had three cases of gastric obstruction following fundoplication and hiatoplasty secondary to the wrap migration into the thorax. Reoperation consisted of reduction of the herniated stomach into the abdomen, mesh-reinforced hiatoplasty and refundoplication.

Lastly, in one case of early occlusion in a patient having undergone gastric resection caused by stenosis of the transmesocolic efferent loop resulting from pancreatitis, conversion in laparotomy was required due to the extreme fixation of the efferent loop. The treatment in this case consisted in a Billroth's operation II.

To evaluate the results of our series on the laparoscopic treatment of complications after surgical or endoscopic procedures, we considered the following items: timing of reoperation, operative time, conversion rate, hospital stay, morbidity and mortality (Table 13.3).

The procedure was successfully carried out by laparoscopy in 158 patients (98.7%). In cases of bleeding reoperation was performed after 14.3 hours (mean, range 0.5–58 hours), with a mean operative time of 45 minutes (range 23-75 minutes). The conversion rate was 0. Patients with peritonitis had reoperation after 55.6 hours (mean, range 38–121 hours), with a mean operative time of 86 minutes (range 55–166 minutes). Reoperation for bowel obstruction was performed after 74 hours (mean, range 48–130 hours), with a mean operation time of 63 minutes (range 47–121 minutes). The conversion rate was 4%.

The overall postoperative hospital stay was 4.9 days (range 3–12 days); it was longer for patients with generalized peritonitis III-IV degree according to

Table 13.3 Outcome

	Bleeding	Peritonitis	Obstruction
Timing of relaparascopy and range (h)	14.3 (0.5–58)	55.6 (38–121)	74 (48–130)
Mean operative time and range (min)	45 (23–75)	86 (55–166)	63 (47–121)
Conversion rate (%)	0	1.2	4
Postoperative stay and range (days)	3.1 (2–5)	8.2 (6–12)	4.2 (2–7)
Postoperative complications (%)	1.14	6.81	16
Mortality (%)	0	2.56	4

Hinchey classification (mean 8.2 days, range 6–12 days) than for patients with bowel obstruction (mean 4.2 days, range 2–7 days) and bleeding (mean 3.1 days, range 2–5 days).

The overall morbidity rate in our series was 7.5% (12/160). Complications included four cases of subphrenic abscess treated with percutaneous CT-guided drainage, four cases of respiratory failure due to bronchopneumonia associated with pleural effusion, treated with medical therapy and thoracentesis in one case, two cases of pulmonary embolism treated with conservative medical therapy, two cases of heart failure treated with medical therapy.

The mortality rate in our series was 1.87%. Three patients died: one died from myocardial infarction on the 15th postoperative day, after discharge in good general conditions, one died from pulmonary embolism on the thent postoperative day and another died from sepsis on the 18th postoperative day.

13.3.3 Discussion

Since its introduction, laparoscopy has undergone constant evolution, which has led it to become the gold standard for surgical treatment in an increasing number of diseases. Laparoscopy has been an important diagnostic tool since the beginning of 20th century and still today it is useful for the correct planning of many medical and surgical treatments [1].

Thanks to the refinement of techniques, the growing experience of surgeons and the diffusion of highly specialized centers, the laparoscopic approach has gradually gained importance in the diagnosis and treatment of emergencies, showing the advantages it has already demonstrated in elective surgery compared to open surgery.

In the emergency setting, the laparoscopic approach should be considered a valid option when noninvasive diagnostic tools are insufficient or give uncertain results [14], because it provides a direct and optimal vision of the entire abdominal cavity, allowing an accurate diagnosis to be made and even proper treatment with minimal trauma for the patient, thus avoiding laparotomy [3].

In a series of 55 patients with acute abdomen, Chung et al. [9] demonstrated that the diagnostic accuracy of laparoscopy is equal to that of laparotomy. Kirshtein et al. [15] report that laparoscopy provides a correct diagnosis in 98.6% of patients with acute abdomen. Many series report a diagnostic benefit of laparoscopy ranging from 89% to 100% [23–25].

Published data clearly confirm the efficacy and safety of laparoscopy as a valid diagnostic and therapeutic option even in emergencies; in fact it contributes to the management of 80% of cases of acute abdomen [9, 26]. Abdominal emergencies are often a diagnostic challenge for the surgeon, as many different diseases may have the same clinical presentation, so a correct diagnosis and an adequate treatment become crucial [10, 27, 28]. In cases of peritonitis, laparoscopy allows a complete exploration of the abdominal cavity, with good lavage of the abdominal recesses [1, 23].

However, still today some authors consider peritonitis a contraindication to laparoscopy, because of the increased risk of bacteremia and endotoxinemia which could be caused by pneumoperitoneum [10–12, 14, 29]. Although concern exists about the use of laparoscopy in cases of peritonitis, on the basis of our experience and in agreement with some authors we believe that the laparoscopic approach is safe and effective in such cases [10, 24, 30–39].

13.4 Conclusions

Based on our experience, we suggest the laparoscopic approach for the treatment of endoscopic and surgical postoperative complications, as it is safe and efficient, although sometimes difficult. Laparoscopic exploration preserves abdominal wall integrity, provides complete visualization of the abdominal cavity and quick identification of the complication, thus allowing good management and resolution. Moreover, laparoscopic surgery reduces mortality, morbidity and hospital stay and improves the quality of life of the patient with fast recovery, less pain and early return to daily activities.

References

1. Kirshtein B, Roy-Shapira A, Lantsberg L et al (2003) The use of laparoscopy in abdominal emergencies. Surg End 17:1118-1124
2. Kirshtein B, Roy-Shapira A, Domchik S et al (2008) Early laparoscopy for management of suspected postoperative complications. J Gastrointest Surg 12:1257-1262
3. Schrenk P, Woisetschlager R, Rieger R, Wayand W (1996) Mechanism management, and prevention of laparoscopic bowel injuries. Gastrointest Endosc 43:572-574
4. Schafer M, Lauper M, Krahenbuhl L (2001) Trocar and Veres needle injuries during laparoscopy. Surg End 15:275-280
5. Shamiyeh A, Wayand W (2004) Laparoscopic cholecystectomy: early and late complications and their treatment. Langenbecks Arch Surg 389:164-171
6. Papasavas PK, Caushaj PF, McCormick JT et al (2003) Laparoscopic management of complications following laparoscopic Roux-en-Y gastric bypass for morbid obesity. Surg End 17:610-614

7. Perrone JM, Soper NJ, Eagon JC et al (2005) Perioperative outcomes and complications of laparoscopic ventral hernia repair. Surgery 138:708-715
8. Dexter SP, Miller GV, Davides D et al (2000) Relaparoscopy for the detection and treatment of complications of laparoscopic cholecystectomy. Am J Surg 179:316-319
9. Chung RS, Diaz JJ, Chari V (1998) Efficacy of routine laparoscopy for the acute abdomen. Surg End 12:219-222
10. Agresta F, Ciardo LF, Mazzarolo G et al (2006) Peritonitis: laparoscopic approach. World J Emerg Surg 1:9
11. Agresta F, De Simone P, Bedin N (2004) The laparoscopic approach in abdominal emergencies. A single-center 10-year experience. JSLS 8:25-30
12. Agresta F, Michelet I, Colucci G, Bedin N (2000) Emergency laparoscopy. A community hospital experience. Surg End 14:154-156
13. Branicki FJ (2002) Abdominal emergencies: diagnostic and therapeutic laparoscopy. Surg Infect (Larchmt) 3:269-282
14. Sauerlenad S, Agresta F, Bergamaschi R et al (2006) Laparoscopy for abdominal emergencies: evidence based guidelines of the European Association for Endoscopic Surgery. Surg End 20:14-29
15. Kirshtein B, Domchik S, Mizrahi S et al (2009) Laparoscopic diagnosis and treatment of postoperative complications. Am J Surg 197:19-23
16. Rosin D, Zmora O, Khaikin M et al (2004) Laparoscopic management of surgical complications after a recent laparotomy. Surg End 18:994-996
17. Tracey D, Arnell MD (2006) Minimally invasive reoperation following laparotomy. Clin Colon Rectal Surg 19:223-227
18. Corcione F, Tricarico F, Barbaros U et al (2008) Gastric volvulus after laparoscopic left adrenalectomy: case report. Surg Laparosc Endosc Percutan Tech 18:207-208
19. Lau WY, Leung KL, Zhu XL et al (1995) Laparoscopic repair of perforated peptic ulcer. Br J Surg 82:814-816
20. So JBY, Kum CK, Fernandes ML, Goh P (1996) Comparison between laparoscopic and conventional omental patch repair for perforated duodenal ulcer. Surg End 10:1060-1063
21. Ibrahim IM, Wolodiger F, Sussman B et al (1996) Laparoscopic management of acute small bowel obstruction. Surg End 10:1012-1015
22. Corcione F, Miranda L, Settembre A et al (2007) Open Veress assisted technique. Results in 2700 cases. Minerva Chir 62:443-446
23. Cuesta MA, Eijsbouts QAJ, Gordijn RV et al (1998) Diagnostic laparoscopy in patients with an acute abdomen of uncertain etiology. Surg End 12:915-917
24. Sanna A, Adani GL, Anania G, Donini A (2003) The role of laparoscopy in patients with suspected peritonitis: experience of a single institution. J Laparoendosc Adv Surg Tech A 13:17-19
25. Geis WP, Kim HC (1995) Use of laparoscopy in the diagnosis and treatment of patients with surgical abdominal sepsis. Surg End 9:178-182
26. Vander Velpen GC, Shimi SM, Cuschieri A (1994) Diagnostic yield and management benefit of laparoscopy: a prospective audit. Gut 35:1617-1621
27. Udwadia TE (2004) Diagnostic laparoscopy. A 30-year overview. Surg End 18:6-10
28. Vons C (1999) Laparoscopy with a diagnostic aim in abdominal emergencies. Chirurgie 124:182-186
29. Neudecker J, Sauerland S, Neugebaur E et al (2002) The European Association for Endoscopic Surgery clinical practice guideline on the pneumoperitoneum for laparoscopic surgery. Surg End 16:1121-1143
30. Farooq A, Ammori BJ (2005) Laparoscopic diagnosis and management of primary bacterial peritonitis. Surg Laparosc Endosc Percutan Tech 15:36-37
31. Heinzelmann M, Schob O, Gianom D et al (1999) Role of laparoscopy in the management of acute appendicitis. Zetralbl Chir 124:1130-1136
32. Kald A, Kullman E, Anderberg B et al (1999) Cost minimization of laparoscopic and open appendectomy. Eur J Surg 165:579-582

33. Lau H (2004) Laparoscopic repair of perforated peptic ulcer. Surg End 18:1013-1021
34. Mancini GJ, Mancini ML, Nelson HS (2005) Efficacy of laparoscopic appendectomy in appendicitis with peritonitis. Am Surg 71:1-4
35. Navez B, Mutter D, Russier Y et al (2001) Safety of laparoscopic approach for acute cholecystitis: retrospective study of 609 cases. World J Surg 2:1352-1356
36. Navez B, Tassetti V, Scohy JJ et al (1998) Laparoscopic management of acute peritonitis. Br J Surg 85:32-36
37. Paya K, Rauhofer U, Rebhandl W et al (2000) Perforating appendicitis. An indication for laparoscopy? Surg End 14:182-184
38. Ramachandran CS, Agarwal S, Dip DG, Arora V (2004) Laparoscopic surgical management of perforative peritonitis in enteric fever. A preliminary study. Surg Laparosc Endosc Percutan Tech 14:122-124
39. Siu WT, Chau CH, Law BKB et al (2004) Routine use of laparoscopic repair for perforated peptic ulcer. Br J Surg 91:481-484

Suggested Readings

Sauerland S, Agresta F, Bergamaschi R, Borzellino G, Budzynski A, Champault G, Fingerhut A, Isla A, Johansson M, Lundorff P (2006) Laparoscopy for abdominal emergencies. Evidence-based guidelines of the European Association for Endoscopic Surgery. Surg Endosc 20:14–29

Agresta F, Ansaloni L, Baiocchi L, Bergamini C, Campanile FB, Carlucci M, Cocorullo G, Corradi A, Franzato B, Lupo M, Mandalà V, Mirabella A, Pernazza G, Piccoli M, Staudacher C, Vettoretto N, Zago M, Lettieri E, Levati A, Pietrini D, Scaglione M, De Masi S, De Placido G, Francucci M, Rasi M, Scaramuzza G, Del Favero AL (2011) Consensus Development Conference of the Società Italiana Chirurgia Endoscopica e nuove tecnologie (SICE); Associazione Chirurghi Ospedalieri Italiani (ACOI); Società Italiana di Chirurgia (SIC); Società Italiana Chirurgia d'Urgenza e Trauma (SICUT), Società Italiana Chirurghi dell'Ospedalità Privata (SICOP) and the European Association for Endoscopic Surgery (EAES). In press

Abdominal Trauma and Laparoscopy

14

Vincenzo Mandalà, Massimo Lupo, Antonino Mirabella
and Benedetto La Motta

14.1 Introduction

Laparoscopy has seen considerable progress in recent years; so it is not surprising that its application has been recommended in all abdominal emergencies, whether traumatic or nontraumatic. In truth the idea of a service of minimally invasive surgery began to be used in abdominal emergencies long before laparoscopy really emerged as a surgical technique. In fact since the 1920s peritoneoscopy or coelioscopy was postulated for diagnosing traumatic hemoperitoneum [1, 2].

In 1941, laparoscopy was considered contraindicated for stab wounds, gunshot wounds and acute viscus perforation out of fear of spreading infection [3]. As early as 1970, Heselson reported the nonoperative treatment of penetrating abdominal injuries, which he explored laparoscopically [4].

After this small series, in 1976, Gazzaniga et al. [5] published a study of 37 patients with abdominal trauma. Three of those patients with penetrating injuries were successfully treated nonoperatively after laparoscopic examination. The problem, then, was essentially the same as it is now: *the diagnostic dilemma of deciding whether a laparotomy should be performed* [9].

The fear of missing an injury and the low quality of instruments and technology led to increased exploration whenever there was any doubt about the findings. At the time, it was thought that the surgical trauma need not be taken into consideration. With trauma laparotomies, as well as with musculoskeletal injuries, the first commandment for trauma surgery was the definitive treatment of all injuries.

Only the long-term analysis of treatment approach tactic has shown that

V. Mandalà (✉)
Department of General and Emergency Surgery,
"Villa Sofia – Cervello" Hospital Trust, Palermo, Italy

V. Mandalà, *The Role of Laparoscopy in Emergency Abdominal Surgery*,

the outcome depends not only on the injury pattern, but also on the treatment strategy. It has become clear that a negative laparotomy carries the risk of increased morbidity and mortality, and that minimally invasive procedures significantly reduce the additional surgical trauma or, in the case of negative laparotomies, avoid it entirely.

In spite of the developments in imaging modalities in the last 30 years, peritoneal penetration with stab wounds as well as injuries to the diaphragm and intestinal tract can confront the surgeon with difficult decisions; here, diagnostic thoracoscopy or laparoscopy can provide decisive information. A further advantage of minimally invasive surgery is that, in unclear cases, laparoscopic exploration can prevent delays in providing definitive treatment. In cases presenting with vague symptoms where the choice to perform an invasive exploration via laparotomy is difficult, the option of less invasive laparoscopic exploration can be attractive [6].

Laparoscopy, only in patients with hemodynamic stability, is, however, valuable not only for its diagnostic but also for its therapeutic potential. Mesenterial tears, as well as some injuries to hollow viscus, parenchymatous organs and the diaphragm, can be repaired quickly and safely, with less stress imposed on the patient [7-9].

14.2 Indications

The range of applications for laparoscopy has greatly expanded with technical advances and the constantly increasing experience with it in acute care surgery, including trauma surgery. Trauma centers throughout the world have developed their own algorithms for handling blunt and penetrating abdominal trauma to assure the fast and effective diagnosis of visceral injuries.

Also today the usual diagnostic procedures of diagnostic peritoneal lavage (DPL), sonography and CT all have their strengths and weaknesses, and none of them are 100% reliable. For this reason, exploratory laparotomy is often performed in the case of stab wounds, but the associated morbidity can reach up to 40% [10].

Diagnostic Laparoscopy (DL) is indicated in hemodynamically stable patients (and in the absence of general absolute contraindications) with suspected intra-abdominal lesions and equivocal findings on imaging studies and when nonoperative management (NOM) is not indicated (suspected hollow viscus injuries with peritonitis, potential diaphragmatic lesion) (EL 1b) [11-13]. The procedure has been shown to effectively decrease the rate of negative laparotomies and the observation time and minimize patient morbidity [14, 15]. The sensitivity, specificity, and accuracy of diagnostic laparoscopy (DL) used to predict the need for laparotomy are high (75% to 100%) (EL 1b) [11, 16, 17], but depend on several factors. The use of DL for trauma is reported to avoid a median 57% (range 17–89%) of patients a nontherapeutic laparotomy (EL 1b) [11, 18, 19].

Table 14.1 Indications for laparoscopy in trauma in hemodynamically stable patients

Blunt abdominal trauma (EL 4) [8]
Penetrating trauma of the abdomen with documented or equivocal penetration of the anterior fascia;
Penetrating thoracoabdominal trauma
Abdominal gunshot wounds with doubtful intraperitoneal trajectory (tangential gunshot wounds) [13, 14]
Suspected diaphragmatic injury, in which imaging occult injury rates are significant, it offers the best diagnostic accuracy
NOM with a progressive worsening of clinical, laboratory and imaging data, but always in presence of hemodynamic stability

Modified from [25]. *NOM*, Nonoperative Management.

The main benefits of laparoscopy are that it can reduce the rate of nontherapeutic and negative laparotomies, identify diaphragmatic injuries accurately, and, in some cases, provide a therapeutic option. It should be emphasized that the use of laparoscopy in patients with trauma is reserved for hemodynamically stable patients and that laparoscopy can have limitations in dorsal stab injuries to the hollow viscus.

The opinion in the early 1990s, supported by published data, that there was a higher incidence of complications with laparoscopy is now outdated, due to increasing experience and technical improvements [8]. The most common indications for laparoscopic diagnosis and treatment in trauma are summarized in Table 14.1.

Another indication is in the some trauma patients who have had free blood fluid diagnosed in the peritoneal cavity, but the source of bleeding cannot be determined. In these patients, nonoperative treatment is usually a risky option. The source is mostly a mesenteric laceration which will often be missed with CT scanning and detected laparoscopically [9].

14.2.1 Blunt Trauma

In our opinion, the most complete description regarding the planning and indications for blunt trauma was provided Selman Uranüs in 2010. This classification was modified by us according to our own personal experience and other data in the literature.

- *Hemoperitoneum with slow and steady increase, with overt parenchymal injury and haemodinamic stability*. In these cases there will be a gradual fall in blood parameters during nonoperative management (NOM), as pointed out by Velmahos in 2003 [46].
- In such *suspected intraperitoneal injury* laparoscopy can provide a certain diagnosis with therapeutic potential (suturing over the laceration or resection).

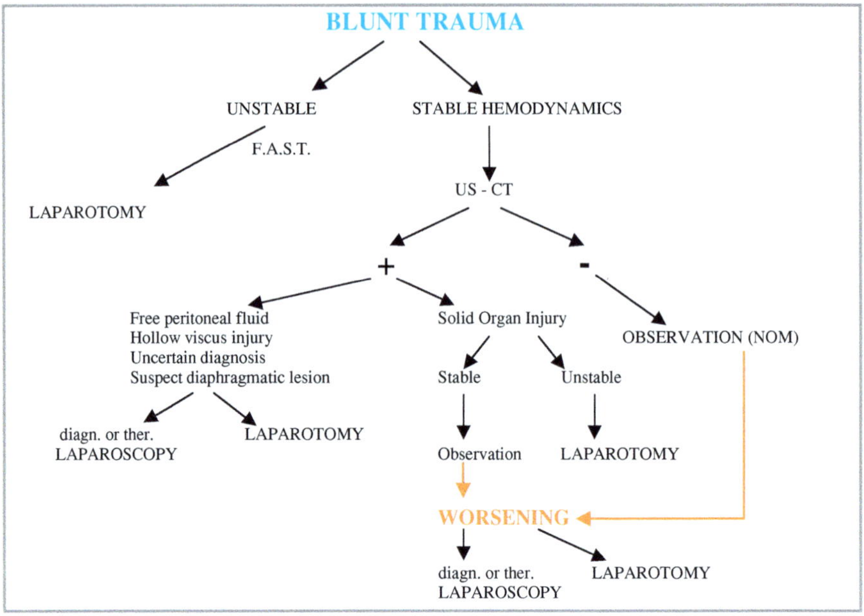

Fig. 14.1 Algorithm for laparoscopy in abdominal blunt trauma. Flowchart by V. Mandalà, 2011

- *Injury to the mesentery, unclear vascular damage to the intestine*. The presence of mesenteric hematoma or lacerations, particularly if there is active bleeding, showed at CT angiography in stable patients, is an indication for diagnostic and/or therapeutic laparoscopy (Figs. 14.1, 14.2). This approach, as well as control of bleeding, may a possible visceral segment identify ischemic and indicate the right treatment (Figs. 14.3-14.8).
- *Unclear abdomen after blunt trauma*. The term *unclear abdomen* indicates a discrepancy between the findings of imaging studies and clinical examination. In spite of conservative treatment, the patient is faced with a worsening of symptoms, which in these conditions are due to conditions not related to the trauma. Laparoscopy can quickly clarify such situations and may also provide a therapeutic option.
- *Pancreatic injury* should be reserved for superficial lesions and without ductal involvement in a proper diagnostic laparoscopy, which requires a broad view of the lesser sac and then of the pancreas. For this method preoperative guidance through imaging is essential and intraoperative ultrasonography is mandatory.

14.2.2 Penetrating Trauma

- *Stable patient with stab wounds*. Laparoscopy allows the diagnosis of peritoneal penetration and subsequent exploration for other organ injuries.

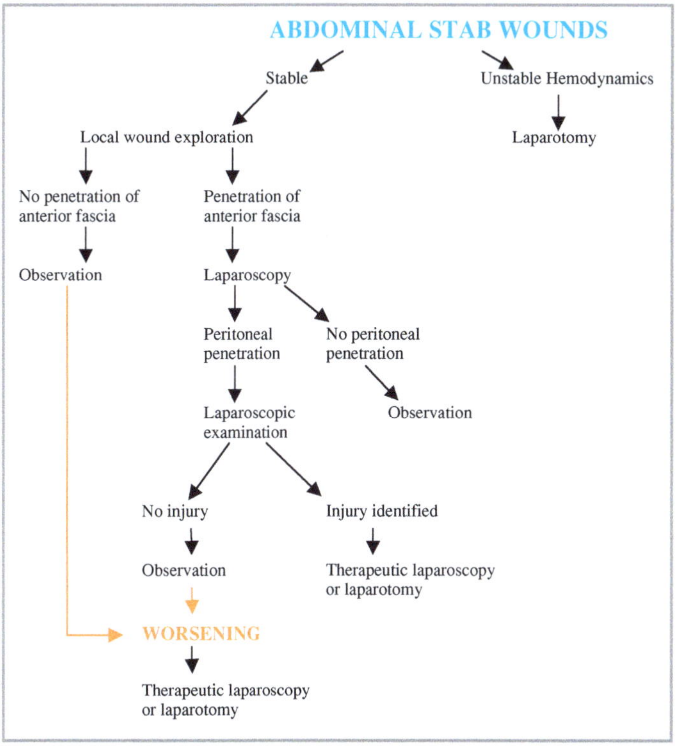

Fig. 14.2 Algorithm for laparoscopy in abdominal stab wound. Flowchart by V. Mandalà, 2011

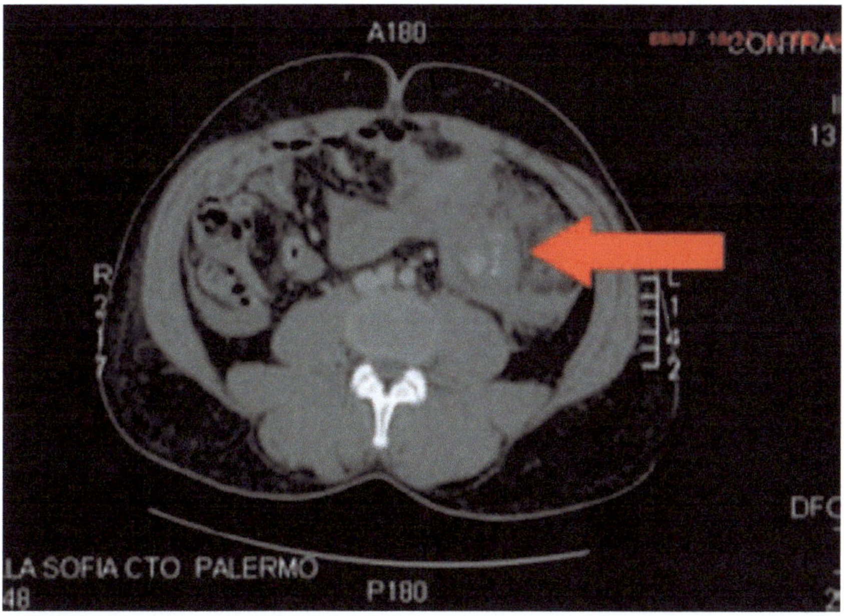

Fig. 14.3 Mesosigmoid blunt traumatic rupture. CT scan: active bleeding (blush in mesosigmoid) (*arrow*)

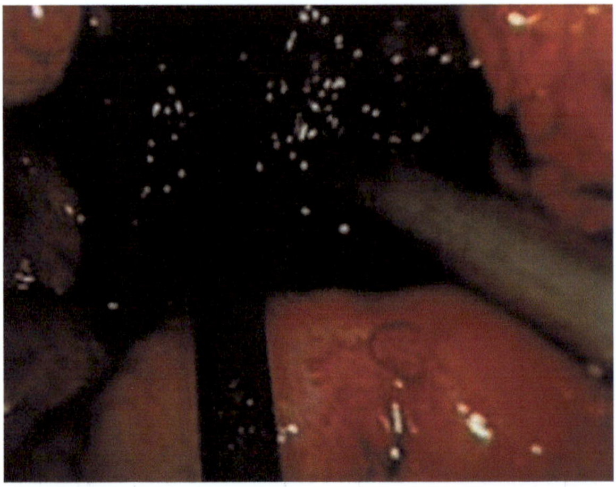

Fig. 14.4 Mesosigmoidal hematoma diagnosed by laparoscopy. Removal of the clots

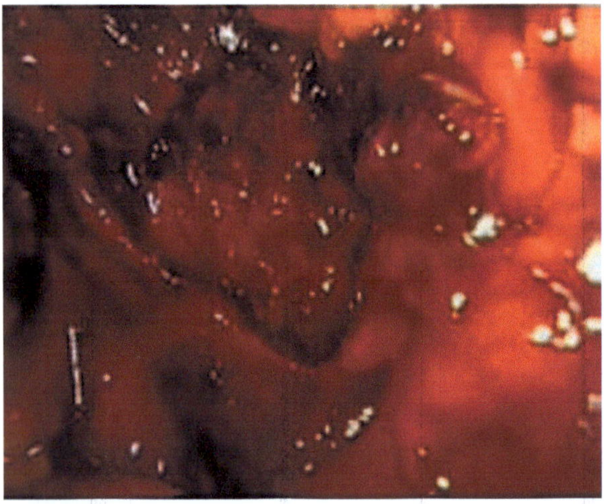

Fig. 14.5 After removing the clots, active bleeding from mesosigmoid vessels is visible

Depending on the severity, the laparoscopic treatment of organ injuries such as those to the stomach wall or intestine may be possible.

- *Diagonal thoracoabdominal stab wounds*: All recent studies conclude that laparoscopy has an important role in this field. This approach to intrathoracic abdominal wounds is strongly indicated to reveal diaphragmatic lesions (coupled with thoracoscopy) (Figs. 14.9-14.12).
- *Gunshot wounds in the flank (tangential gunshot)*. For gunshot wounds, laparoscopy can be used as a means of triage to rule out peritoneal violation in selected cases when the clinical examination is equivocal. Sosa et al. [15, 16] selected hemodynamically stable patients with wounds in which the path of the bullet appeared tangential to the peritoneal cavity.

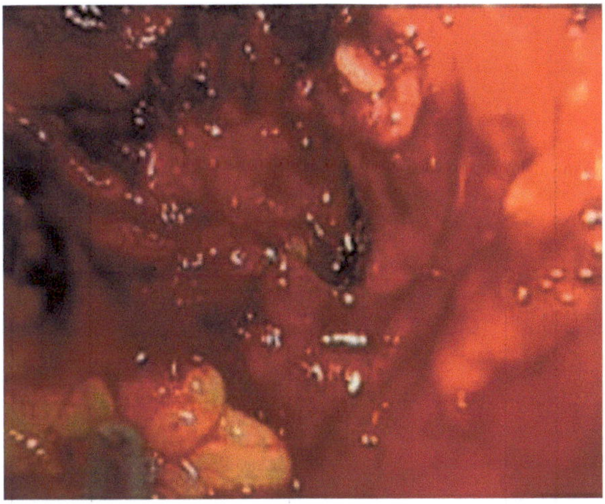

Fig. 14.6 Bleeding control with clips and floseal

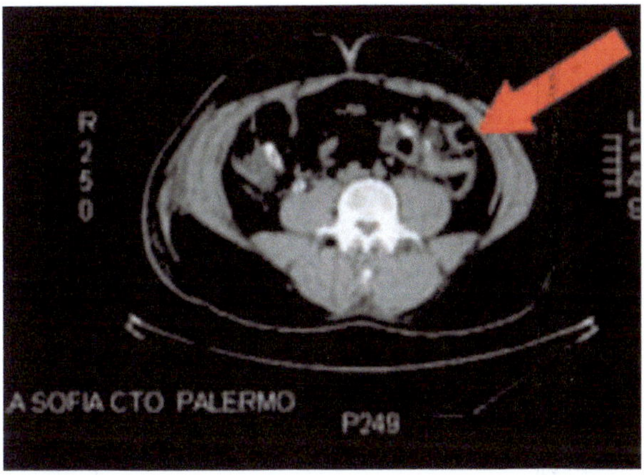

Fig. 14.7 Follow-up with CT scan

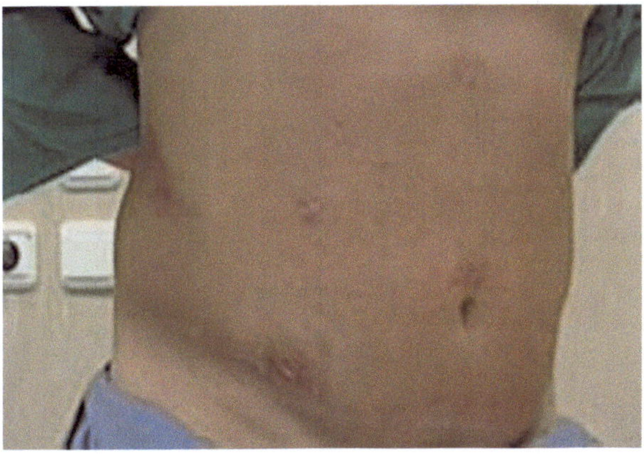

Fig. 14.8 Follow-up one month later. Abdominal wall

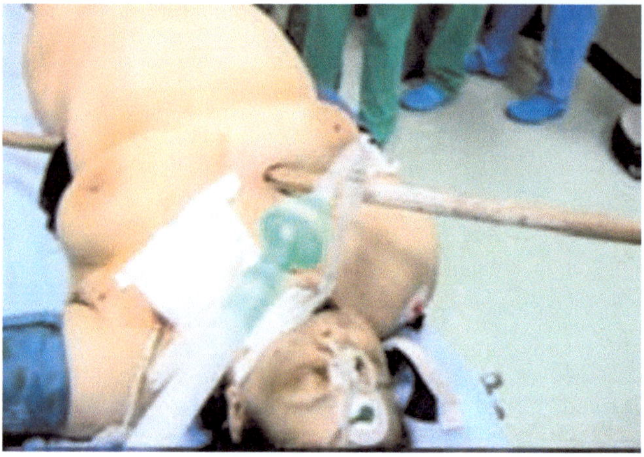

Fig. 14.9 A 42-year-old female patient, fallen from the first floor, impaled. Stable hemodynamic conditions. Negative CT for abdominal effusion, free air, etc.

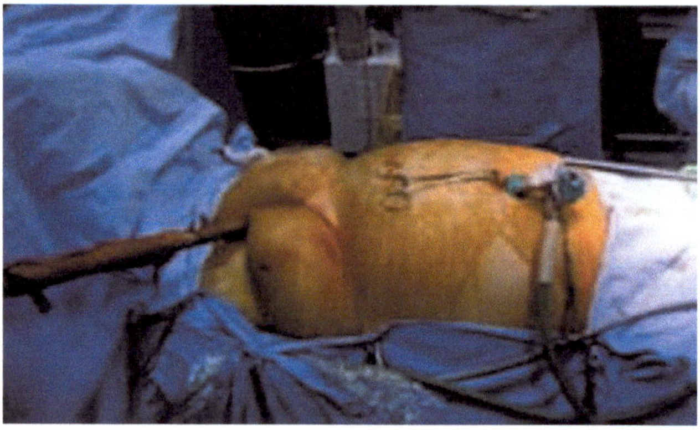

Fig. 14.10 Diagnostic laparoscopy

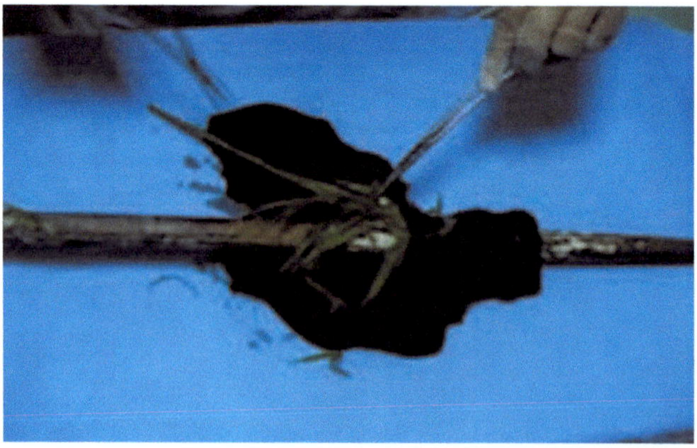

Fig. 14.11 Removal of the pole (pole, cloth and papyrus)

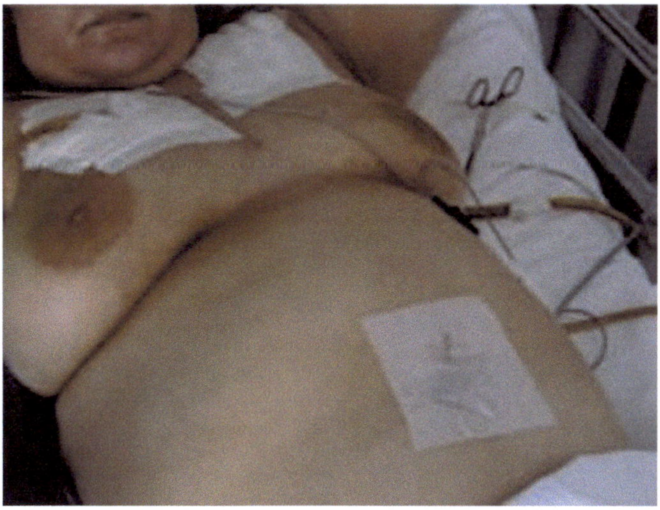

Fig. 14.12 Follow-up two days after surgery. Discharge on the fifth day

Ortega et al. [17] described the advantages of laparoscopy for stabbed abdomens. Laparoscopy avoids unnecessary laparotomy and prevents the risk of undiagnosed hollow viscus injury leading to delayed laparotomy for acute peritonitis.

- *Suspected diaphragmatic injury*. A thoraco-abdominal CT or MR diagnosis may miss an injury to the diaphragm, because a viscous shift from the abdomen to the thorax could occur subsequently (today even some cases are diagnosed only at autopsy): in these cases the wound can be explored laparoscopically or thoracoscopically to determine whether laparotomy, thoracotomy, or a minimal access procedure is indicated.

14.3 Technique

Success can very much depend on the correct choice of trocar positions. For therapeutic maneuvers, the triangulation of the area of injury is immensely important for intracorporeal sewing and suturing. Organs can be shifted by changing the position of the operating table so that the surgical field can be better visualized without additional trocars and retractors (Fig. 14.13).

The procedure is usually performed under general anesthesia; however, local anesthesia with I.V. sedation has also been used successfully in the emergency department (awake laparoscopy) (EL 3) [20-26]. We are convinced that general anesthesia in the operating room is the best option because it allows an in - depth examination (multiple positions) and therapeutic possibilities, whereas the awake laparoscopy in the emergency room with mini optical involves, in our opinion, a perfunctory examination.

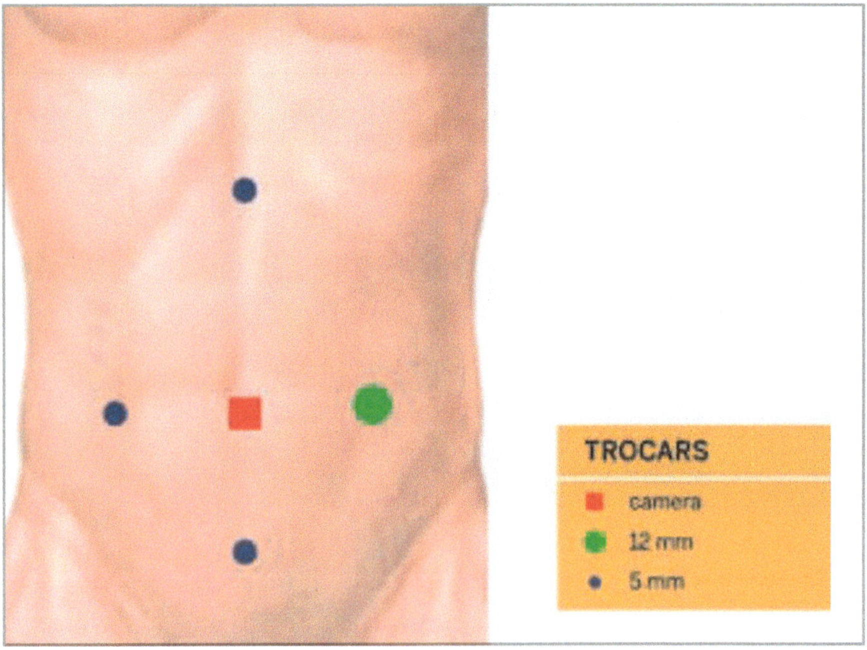

Fig. 14.13 Choice of trocar site for diagnostic laparoscopy in trauma. The image shows the umbilical port for the laparoscope, additional ports (lateral to muscle) for the operation. The epigastric port and the suprapubic port are optional (5 mm or 10 mm trocars)

Many authors have used low insufflation pressures (8-12 mmHg); however, pressures up to 15 mmHg have been described without untoward events [23]. Special attention should be given to the possibility of a tension pneumothorax caused by the pneumoperitoneum due to an unsuspected diaphragmatic rupture. The pneumoperitoneum is created usually through a periumbilical incision using an open technique or a Veress needle assisted technique in the left hypocondrium, after insertion of a nasogastric tube and a Foley catheter.

A 30-degree laparoscope is advantageous; diagnostic exploration for peritoneal penetration or diaphragmatic injury could be performed using a single camera port and additional trocars are used for organ manipulations. In the case of penetrating wounds, air leaks can be controlled with sutures. The peritoneal cavity can be examined systematically, beginning with the right upper quadrant and proceeding clockwise, taking advantage of patient positioning manipulations. Suction/irrigation may be needed for optimal visualization, and methylene blue can be administered intravenously or via a nasogastric tube to help identify urologic or stomach injuries, respectively [24]. The colon can be mobilized and the lesser sac inspected. After a thorough exploration, if a hollow viscus lesions has not been found, blood can be vacuumed off into a Cell Saver® for autotrasfusion (EL 3b) [19, 25-27].

In penetrating injuries, peritoneal violation can be determined [23]. It must be kept in mind that it is easy to miss small bowel perforations and retroperitoneal injuries to the colon [19].

The surgeon should not hesitate to do an exploratory laparotomy if he or she is not 100% certain that there are no missed injuries (EL 3) [19].

14.4 Therapeutic Laparoscopy

In a highly selected group of patients therapeutic laparoscopy should be performed only by surgeons skilled in advanced mini-invasive surgery (EL 3a) [19, 28]. Its use in blunt trauma is more limited but appears applicable for some patients requiring operative repair of other injuries (EL 2a) [29]. Bleeding from minor injuries of the liver or the spleen can be controlled through the laparoscope (EL 4) [30, 31].

Therapeutic laparoscopic options have broadened in recent years to include hemoperitoneum as well as mesentery and hollow viscus injuries [25] (hemostasis of minor bleeding and minor visceral injuries), but especially for diaphragmatic laparoscopic repair of small and isolated injuries and to avoid in most cases non-therapeutic laparotomy. Diaphragmatic lacerations (EL 4) [32-34] and perforating stab wounds of the gastrointestinal tract can be sewn or stapled safely when laparoscopic expertise is available (EL 4) [19, 20, 35].

Angiographic embolization is an acceptable option to further define and treat splenic and liver injuries in hemodynamically stable patients to reduce the rate of observation (NOM) and surgical intervention (EL 4) [36, 37].

No attempt to repair complex injuries laparoscopically should be made, because the potential benefits of the minimally invasive approach do not outweigh the risk [38].

In some referral centers delayed laparoscopy is proposed as a valid diagnostic and therapeutic means (EL 4) [39, 40], especially for hepatic related complications usually consisting of bleeding biliary, hepatic abscess or necrosis and development of abdominal compartment syndrome [28, 41, 42]. Thus laparoscopy should not be considered a failure of NOM, but a part of this therapeutic strategy coupled with radiologic and endoscopic interventional procedures.

14.5 Limitations and Complications of Laparoscopy for Trauma

With regard to the inclusion of laparoscopy in the diagnostic algorithm, critics or non-supporters of the technique have always stressed its limitations: invasiveness, considerable costs and associated complications. There are organizational limitations regarding the need to have an operating room available around the clock for treating emergencies laparoscopically with trained personnel and all the ancillary services (radiology, ultrasonography, transfusion centre and anesthesia), especially at night. There are also the medicolegal implications, especially in terms of informed consent.

14.5.1 Cost Considerations

In a retrospective analysis comparing the total hospital costs of exploratory laparotomy to those of diagnostic laparoscopy in 37 patients with penetrating abdominal trauma, the cost analysis showed that the laparoscopy-based strategy was about EUR 1,136 cheaper than the exploratory laparotomy based strategy (EL 3a) [43]. In a prospective, randomized study of 43 patients with abdominal stab wounds, however, there was no difference between the two strategies in the total hospital costs (EL 1b) [11].

14.5.2 Complications

The complications may be inherent to the technique, and trauma related. Complications of laparoscopy related to trauma include not only the usual complications of anesthesia and laparoscopy, but also procedure-related complications. They occur in up to 11% of patients and are usually minor (EL 1b) [7, 11, 19, 29]. Recent studies report a median of 0 (0-10%) morbidity and 0% mortality (EL 1b) [11, 19, 35, 44, 45]. Complications include:

- tension pneumothorax in patients with diaphragmatic injury from positive-pressure pneumoperitoneum [20, 7];
- gas embolism in patients with intra-abdominal venous injuries, especially in liver;
- lacerations (role of *gasless* laparoscopy).

The transperitoneal absorption of carbon dioxide may cause metabolic and hemodynamic changes such as acidosis, cardiac suppression, atelectasis, subcutaneous emphysema and increased intracranial pressure, resulting in more profound consequences for the trauma patient.

Perforation of a hollow viscus, laceration of a solid organ, vascular injury (usually trocar injury of an epigastric artery or lacerated omental vessels), and subcutaneous or extraperitoneal dissection by the insufflation of gas may also occur. Port-site infections may occur during the postoperative course.

14.6 Conclusions

In recent years, more so then in the past, it seems more justified to widen the indications for laparoscopy in abdominal trauma. A more rigorous surgical strategy requires that surgeons consider the laparoscopic approach to be an important tool in their hands, and that they use this approach in a rational way in well codified situations, in well organized and dedicated centers. However, in our opinion, the best indication remains a suspected peritoneal tear in hemodynamically stable patients.

We believe that in several other cases, strictly in the operating room, an explorative laparoscopy can be performed instead of a mandatory laparotomy.

Today therapeutic laparoscopy can be undertaken in an increasing number of cases, based on the reported evidence, common sense and right skill, to achieve a synergy and not a conflict between evidence based medicine and daily practice.

References

1. Short AR (1925) The use of coelioscopy. BMJ 2:254-255
2. Stone WE (1924) Intra-abdominal examination by the aid of the peritoneoscope. J Kansas Med Soc 24:63-65
3. Beling CA (1941) Selection of cases for peritoneoscopy. Arch Surg 42:872-889
4. Heselson J (1970) Peritoneoscopy in abdominal trauma. S Afr J Surg 8:53-61
5. Gazzaniga AB, Stanton WW, Bartlett RH (1976) Laparoscopy in the diagnosis of blunt and penetrating injuries to the abdomen. Am J Surg 131:315-318
6. Murray JA, Demetriades D, Asensio JA et al (1998) Occult injuries to the diaphragm: prospective evaluation of laparoscopy in penetrating injuries to the left lower chest. J Am Coll Surg 187:626-630
7. Ivatury RR, Simon RJ, Stahl WM (1993) A critical evaluation of laparoscopy in penetrating abdominal trauma. J Trauma 34:822-828
8. Villavicencio RT, Aucar JA (1999) Analysis of laparoscopy in trauma. J Am Coll Surg 189:11-20
9. Uranüs S (2010) Minimally invasive surgery in trauma and emergencies. Eur J Trauma Emerg Surg 36:1
10. Uranüs S, Dorr K (2010) Laparoscopy in abdominal trauma. Eur J Trauma Emerg Surg 36:19-24
11. Leppäniemi A, Haapiainen R (2003) Diagnostic laparoscopy in abdominal stab wounds: a prospective, randomized study. J Trauma 55:636-645
12. Cuschieri A, Hennessy T, Stephens RB, Berci G (1988) Diagnosis of significant abdominal trauma after road traffic accidents: preliminary results of a multicentre clinical trial comparing minilaparoscopy with peritoneal lavage. Ann Roy Coll Surg 70:153-155
13. Sauerland S, Agresta F, Bergamaschi R et al (2006) Laparoscopy for abdominal emergencies Evidence-based guidelines of the European Association for Endoscopic Surgery. Surg Endosc 20:14-29
14. Diagnostic Laparoscopy Guidelines: Practice/Clinical Guidelines published on: 11/2007 by the Society of American Gastrointestinal and Endoscopic Surgeons (SAGES)
15. Sosa JL, Arrillaga A, Puente I et al (1995) Laparoscopy in 121 consecutive patients with abdominal gunshot wounds. J Trauma 39:501-506
16. Sosa JL, Baker M, Peunte I et al (1995) Negative laparotomy in abdominal gunshot wounds: potential impact of laparoscopy. J Trauma 38:194-197
17. Ortega AE, Tang E, Froes ET et al (1996) Laparoscopic evaluation of penetrating thoracoabdominal traumatic injuries. Surg Endosc 10:19-22
18. National Guideline Clearinghouse (2009) Diagnostic laparoscopy for trauma. Guideline summary NGC - 6829 (NCG Status: Update information was verified by the guideline developer on March 9, 2009)
19. Choi YB, Lim KS (2003) Therapeutic laparoscopy for abdominal trauma Surg Endosc 17:421-427
20. Mathonnet M, Peyrou P, Gainant A et al (2003) Role of laparoscopy in blunt perforations of the small bowel. Surg Endosc 17:641-645
21. Weinberg JA, Magnotti LJ, Edwards NM et al (2007) “Awake” laparoscopy for the evaluation of equivocal penetrating abdominal wounds”. Injury 38:60-64
22. Berci G, Dunkelman D, Michel SL et al (1983) Emergency minilaparoscopy in abdominal trauma. An update. Am J Surg 146:261-265

23. Stefanidis D, Richardson WS, Lily C et al (2009) The role of diagnostic laparoscopy for acute abdominal conditions: an evidence-based review. Surg Endosc 23:16-23
24. Smith RS, Meister RK, Tsoi EKM et al (1993) Laparoscopically guided blood salvage and autotransfusion in splenic trauma: a case report. J Trauma 34:313-314
25. Zantut LFC, Machado MAC, Volpe P et al (1996) Autotransfusion with laparoscopically salvaged blood in trauma: report on 21 cases. Surg Laparosc Endosc 6:46-48
26. Warren O, Kinross J, Paraskeva P, Darzi A (2006) Emergency laparoscopy - current best practice. World J Emerg Surg 1:24
27. Fabian TC, Croce MA, Stewart RM et al (1993) A prospective analysis of diagnostic laparoscopy in trauma. Ann Surg 217:557-565
28. Chen RJ, Fang JF, Lin BC et al (1998) Selective application of laparoscopy and fibrin glue in the failure of nonoperative management of blunt hepatic trauma. J Trauma 44:691-695
29. Carobbi A, Romagnani F, Antonelli G, Bianchini M (2010) Laparoscopic splenectomy for severe blunt trauma: initial experience of ten consecutive cases with a fast hemostatic technique. Surg Endosc 24:1325-1330
30. Hassanen A, Abou-Bieh H, Nagib Y (2009) Laproscopy for the evaluation of anterior abdominal stab wounds in hemodynamically stable patients. EJS 28:58-61
31. Leppäniemi A, Salo J, Haapiainen R (1995) Complications of negative laparotomy for truncal stab wounds. J Trauma 38:54-58
32. Matthews BD, Bui H, Harold KL et al (2003) Laparoscopic repair of traumatic diaphragmatic injuries. Surg Endosc 17:254-258
33. Smith CH, Novick TL, Jacobs DG, Thomason MH (2000) Laparoscopic repair of a ruptured diaphragm secondary to blunt trauma. Surg Endosc 14:501-502
34. Smith RS, Fry WR, Morabito DJ et al (1995) Therapeutic laparoscopy in trauma. Am J Surg 170:632-637
35. Zantut LF, Ivatury RR, Smith RS et al (1997) Diagnostic and therapeutic laparoscopy for penetrating abdominal trauma: a multicenter experience. J Trauma 42:825-831
36. Sudakoff GS, Yucel EK, Rosen MP et al (2008) Blunt Abdominal Trauma - ACR Appropriateness Criteria®. Available at: http://www.guidelines.gov/content.aspx?id=15726. Accessed 16 June 2011
37. Dissanaike S, Frezza EE (2006) Laparoscopic splenectomy in blunt trauma. JSLS 10:499-503
38. Lin HF, Wu JM, Tu VC Chen H-A, Shih H-C Value of diagnostic and Therapeutic Laparoscopy for Abdominal Stab Wounds. World J Surg (2010) 34: 1653-1662
39. Letoublon C, Chen Y, Arvieux C et al (2008) Delayed celiotomy or laparoscopic as part of the nonoperative management of blunt hepatic trauma. World J Surg 32:1189-1193
40. Marzano E, Rosso E, Oussoultzoglou E et al (2010) Laparoscopic treatment of biliary peritonitis following nonoperative management of blunt liver trauma. World J Emerg Surg 5:26
41. Kozar RA, Moore FA, Cothren CC et al (2006) Risk factors of hepatic morbidity following non operative management: multicenter study. Arch Surg 141:451-458
42. Kozar RA, Moore JB, Niles SE et al(2005) Complications of nonoperative management of blunt hepatic trauma. J Trauma 59:1066-1071
43. Marks JM, Youngelman DF, Berk T (1997) Cost analysis of diagnostic laparoscopy vs laparotomy in the evaluation of penetrating abdominal trauma. Surg Endosc 11:272-276
44. Simon RJ, Rabin J, Kuhls D (2002) Impact of increased use of laparoscopy on negative laparotomy rates after penetrating trauma. J Trauma 53:297-302
45. De Maria EJ, Dalton JM, Gore DC et al (2000) Complementary roles of laparoscopic abdominal exploration and diagnostic peritoneal lavage for evaluating abdominal stab wounds: a prospective study. J Laparoendosc Adv Surg Tech 10:131-136
46. Velmahos GC, Toutouzas KG (2003) Nonoperative treatment of blunt injury to solid abdominal organs: a prospective study. Arch Surg 138:844-851

Suggested Readings

Sauerland S, Agresta F, Bergamaschi R, Borzellino G, Budzynski A, Champault G, Fingerhut A, Isla A, Johansson M, Lundorff P (2006) Laparoscopy for abdominal emergencies. Evidence-based guidelines of the European Association for Endoscopic Surgery. Surg Endosc 20:14–29

Agresta F, Ansaloni L, Baiocchi L, Bergamini C, Campanile FB, Carlucci M, Cocorullo G, Corradi A, Franzato B, Lupo M, Mandalà V, Mirabella A, Pernazza G, Piccoli M, Staudacher C, Vettoretto N, Zago M, Lettieri E, Levati A, Pietrini D, Scaglione M, De Masi S, De Placido G, Francucci M, Rasi M, Scaramuzza G, Del Favero AL (2011) Consensus Development Conference of the Società Italiana Chirurgia Endoscopica e nuove tecnologie (SICE); Associazione Chirurghi Ospedalieri Italiani (ACOI); Società Italiana di Chirurgia (SIC); Società Italiana Chirurgia d'Urgenza e Trauma (SICUT), Società Italiana Chirurghi dell'Ospedalità Privata (SICOP) and the European Association for Endoscopic Surgery (EAES). In press

Subject Index

MIX
Papier aus verantwortungsvollen Quellen
Paper from responsible sources
FSC® C105338

If you have any concerns about our products,
you can contact us on
ProductSafety@springernature.com

In case Publisher is established outside the EU,
the EU authorized representative is:
Springer Nature Customer Service Center GmbH
Europaplatz 3, 69115 Heidelberg, Germany

Printed by Libri Plureos GmbH
in Hamburg, Germany